Synaptic Plasticity - Neurobiology, Neuroanatomy, and Clinical Neuroscience

Edited by Ioannis Mavroudis

Published in London, United Kingdom

Synaptic Plasticity - Neurobiology, Neuroanatomy, and Clinical Neuroscience
http://dx.doi.org/10.5772/intechopen.1003581
Edited by Ioannis Mavroudis

Contributors
Alin Ciobica, CongYu Jin, Dimitrios Kazis, Fenglan Wang, Foivos Petrides, Guiyu Guan, Ioannis Mavroudis, Jiayu Duan, Jun Zhang, Kaj Karlstedt, Katerina Franekova, Mingjun Tan, Piu Chan, Sehyoun Yoon, Shaozhen Ji, Yunling Zhang, Zhongqun Chen

First published in London, United Kingdom, 2025 by IntechOpen
IntechOpen is the global imprint of INTECHOPEN LIMITED, registered in England and Wales, registration number: 11086078, 167-169 Great Portland Street, London, W1W 5PF, United Kingdom

For EU product safety concerns: IN TECH d.o.o., Prolaz Marije Krucifikse Kozulić 3, 51000 Rijeka, Croatia, info@intechopen.com or visit our website at intechopen.com.

British Library Cataloguing-in-Publication Data
A catalogue record for this book is available from the British Library

Synaptic Plasticity - Neurobiology, Neuroanatomy, and Clinical Neuroscience
Edited by Ioannis Mavroudis
p. cm.
Print ISBN 978-1-83634-140-6
Online ISBN 978-1-83634-139-0
eBook (PDF) ISBN 978-1-83634-141-3

Meet the editor

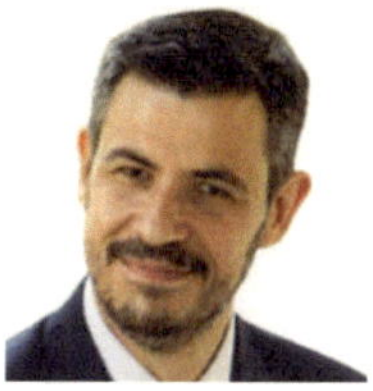

Dr. Ioannis Mavroudis is a consultant neurologist and Senior Lecturer with a special interest in mild traumatic brain injury (mTBI) and neurodegeneration. He holds a Ph.D. in neuropathology and neuromorphology and has been actively involved in research since 2005. Dr. Mavroudis has published over 100 peer-reviewed papers and authored more than eight books in the fields of neurology and neuroscience. With extensive clinical experience, he has worked in traumatic brain injury and has led recovery planning for mTBI patients. He has taught neuroanatomy and neuropathology in Greece, as well as clinical neurology, as a visiting assistant professor at the University of Cyprus. He has also served as a visiting lecturer at the University of Leeds. Recently, he was elected Assistant Professor of Neurology at Aristotle University of Thessaloniki. Dr. Mavroudis is also a leader in medicolegal neurology, providing expert opinions on concussion cases and directing efforts to improve early screening and rehabilitation for head injuries. His work integrates cutting-edge research with practical applications in concussion diagnosis, monitoring, and treatment. As the academic editor of this book, he brings his expertise in both clinical and research aspects of concussions, offering a comprehensive perspective on the subject.

Contents

Preface

Synaptic plasticity—the ability of synapses to strengthen or weaken over time in response to increases or decreases in their activity—is the cornerstone of neurobiological function, from learning and memory to recovery from injury and the development of neuropsychiatric disorders. As our understanding of this fundamental process continues to evolve, it becomes increasingly clear that synaptic plasticity lies at the intersection of molecular biology, structural neuroanatomy, and clinical neuroscience.

This book, *Synaptic Plasticity – Neurobiology, Neuroanatomy, and Clinical Neuroscience*, was conceived to offer a comprehensive and interdisciplinary exploration of the mechanisms, models, and implications of synaptic plasticity. Bringing together contributions from leading scientists, clinicians, and educators, the volume spans a broad spectrum—from molecular mechanisms, such as long-term potentiation and synaptogenesis, to their expression in neuroanatomical pathways and their translation into clinical practice.

The book is structured to serve as both a foundational text and an up-to-date reference. Section I focuses on the molecular and cellular underpinnings of synaptic change, including the roles of neurotransmitters, receptors, and intracellular signaling. Section II delves into the neuroanatomical substrates where plasticity manifests, drawing on both classical and modern brain mapping approaches. Section III connects this knowledge to clinical conditions—such as stroke, epilepsy, neurodegenerative diseases, and psychiatric disorders—highlighting how altered plasticity can inform diagnosis, prognosis, and therapeutic strategies.

Whether you are a neuroscientist, clinician, graduate student, or educator, this book is designed to deepen your understanding of how the brain adapts, learns, and heals. As the editor, I am deeply grateful to the contributors for their intellectual rigor and to the readers for joining us in exploring one of the most dynamic and fascinating realms of modern neuroscience.

Dr. Ioannis Mavroudis
Consultant Neurologist,
Leeds Teaching Hospitals,
NHS Trust,
UK

Honorary Senior Lecturer,
Leeds University,
Leeds, UK

Assistant Professor of Neurology,
Aristotle University of Thessaloniki,
Thessaloniki, Greece

Section 1

Mechanisms of Synaptic Plasticity and Dysfunction

Chapter 1

Pathological Synaptic Plasticity in Neurological Disorders

CongYu Jin and Kaj Karlstedt

Abstract

This chapter will introduce the concept of pathological synaptic plasticity and its pivotal role in the progression of various neurological disorders. Synaptic plasticity, the brain's ability to strengthen or weaken synapses in response to activity, is essential for learning and memory. However, when these mechanisms are disrupted, they can contribute to the pathology of diseases such as Alzheimer's disease, Parkinson's disease, epilepsy, schizophrenia, and autism spectrum disorders. This chapter explores the molecular and cellular foundations of synaptic plasticity, identifies how its dysregulation leads to neurological dysfunction, and examines the clinical implications. Additionally, it reviews current and emerging therapeutic strategies aimed at restoring normal synaptic function, offering insights into potential future research directions and treatment modalities.

Keywords: pathological synaptic plasticity, neurological disorders, synaptic dysfunction, neurodegenerative diseases, neuropsychiatric disorders, therapeutic interventions

1. Introduction

Synaptic plasticity, the ability of synapses to strengthen or weaken over time in response to increases or decreases in their activity [1], is a fundamental property of the brain that underlies essential cognitive processes such as learning, memory, and adaptation to new experiences [2–4]. Synaptic plasticity is achieved through various mechanisms, including long-term potentiation (LTP) [5] and long-term depression (LTD) [6, 7], which involve the modulation of synaptic strength and are critical for maintaining the dynamic functionality of neural circuits.

Aberrations in adaptive changes of synaptic strength and connectivity cause pathological synaptic plasticity, which underlies the development and progress of various neurological disorders such as dementia, Parkinson's disease, and psychiatric disorders. Unlike normal synaptic plasticity that supports healthy brain functions, pathological synaptic plasticity disrupts neuronal communication and can lead to cognitive deficits, behavioral abnormalities, and neurodegeneration. The abnormal plasticity might arise from genetic mutations, environmental stressors, or protein misfolding, and it manifests in various ways in different neurological diseases.

Understanding pathological synaptic plasticity is crucial for several reasons. Firstly, it provides insights into the underlying mechanisms of neurological disorders, which can reveal novel targets for therapeutic intervention. Secondly, it helps in the identification of biomarkers for early diagnosis and monitoring of disease progression. Finally, elucidating the factors that drive pathological changes in synaptic plasticity can support the development of strategies to restore normal synaptic function, thereby improving clinical outcomes for patients with conditions such as Alzheimer's disease, Parkinson's disease, epilepsy, schizophrenia, and autism spectrum disorders.

2. Molecular mechanisms of synaptic plasticity

2.1 Short-term synaptic plasticity

Short-term synaptic plasticity lasts from milliseconds to several minutes and plays important roles in short-term adaptations to sensory inputs, transient changes in behavioral states and short-lasting forms of memory [8]. Most short-term synaptic plasticity is triggered by short burst of activity, which causes a transient accumulation of Ca^{2+} in presynaptic nerve terminals, and modifies biochemical processes underlying exocytosis of synaptic vesicles, thus changing the probability of presynaptic neurotransmitter release.

2.2 N-methyl-D-aspartate receptor (NMDAR)-dependent long-term synaptic plasticity

Long-term synaptic plasticity is activity-dependent and has long-lasting modifications of the synaptic strength. Slow and long-lasting homeostatic processes adjust synaptic strength to maintain circuit activity within functional regimes [9]. Long-term potentiation (LTP) and long-term depression (LTD) are two primary forms of long-term synaptic plasticity that modulate the strength of synaptic connections in the brain.

LTP is the process by which synaptic connections become stronger with repeated stimulation and results in a long-lasting enhancement in synaptic transmission. It is often induced by high-frequency stimulation of synapses and is considered one of the major cellular mechanisms underlying learning and memory [2, 5]. It plays a critical role in memory formation and storage of information in the brain.

Conversely, LTD is the process that weakens synaptic connections and results in a long-lasting decrease in synaptic transmission. It is typically induced by low-frequency stimulation. This weakening helps to eliminate less active synapses, thus refining neural circuits and maintaining synaptic balance. LTD is necessary in preventing the saturation of all synapses and keeping the synaptic selectivity [10]. It plays a crucial role in synaptic pruning, the refinement of neural circuits, and the removal of old memories, making space for new information.

Together, LTP and LTD ensure the plasticity necessary for the adaptive functioning of neural networks that respond constructively to the environmental changes [2, 11].

2.3 Non-NMDAR-dependent LTP

Mossy fiber LTP is another mechanistically distinct form of LTP in the hippocampus that exists at the synapse between the axons of dentate gyrus (DG) granule cells and the dendrites of CA3 pyramidal neurons [12]. It is also found at corticothalamic synapses and cerebellar parallel fiber synapses. Mossy fiber LTP is triggered solely by an activity-dependent rise of intracellular Ca^{2+} level at the presynaptic terminal and the consequent activation of protein kinase A (PKA). It increases the probability of presynaptic neurotransmitter release [2].

2.4 Non-NMDAR-dependent LTD

The induction of metabotropic glutamate receptor (mGluR)-dependent LTD requires the activation of extrasynaptic group I mGluRs, namely, mGluR1 and mGluR5 [13]. Cerebellar and ventral tegmental LTD needs activation of mGluR1 and the downstream protein kinase C (PKC) signaling [13–15], while activation of mGluR5 triggers protein tyrosine phosphatase-dependent regulation of postsynaptic expression of α-amino-3-hydroxy-5-methyl-4-isoxazolepropionic acid (AMPA) receptors, contributing to the hippocampal LTD [16]. The mGluR LTD is also dependent on mGluR-triggered protein synthesis [17–20]; however, in neonatal animals, it might involve a retrograde messenger instead of the protein synthesis [8]. The mGluR-dependent LTD at the synapse between parallel fibers and Purkinje cells is also called "cerebellar LTD" [21, 22]. Its induction requires simultaneous activation of parallel fibers and climbing fibers, as well as the coincident activation of mGluR1 and voltage-gated Ca^{2+} channels. The cerebellar LTD reduces the sensitivity of Purkinje cells and is important for certain types of motor learning [8, 23].

In a number of brain regions such as hippocampus, cerebellum, striatum, and cerebral cortex, there exists a type of endocannabinoid-mediated LTD (eCB-LTD). Endocannabinoids are retrograde transmitters released by postsynaptic neurons. Endocannabinoids bind to the presynaptic cannabinoid CB1 receptors, which are abundant and widely distributed in the central nervous system, and activate the Gi/o type of G-protein coupled to them to induce a transient suppress of inhibitory and excitatory synapses via presynaptic reduction or inhibition of GABA or glutamate release [24–29].

2.5 Key molecular players in synaptic plasticity

Given the diversity of the functions ascribed to synaptic plasticity, it is natural that there are various forms of LTP and LTD with different underlying mechanisms in different brain areas [7, 30–32], different neurons [2], and at different ages [33]. Among them, the widely accepted and most extensively studied ones are NMDAR-dependent LTP and LTD. NMDA receptors, AMPA receptors, and calcium signaling are three essential contributors in establishing the NMDAR-dependent LTP. They are also involved in the mechanisms of other types of synaptic plasticities. This section is to provide a foundational understanding of the molecular mechanisms underlying normal synaptic plasticity, focusing on NMDAR-dependent LTP and LTD (for details and other types of plasticity, see relevant chapters in this book).

2.5.1 NMDA receptors

NMDARs are critical for initiating both LTP and LTD. NMDAR is an ionotropic glutamate receptor and its activation requires glutamate binding when the membrane is depolarized [3, 34]. When activated, NMDA ion channels are predominantly permeable to calcium ions (Ca^{2+}) and allow Ca^{2+} influx to enter postsynaptic dendrites, which in turn triggers downstream signaling pathways leading to synaptic strengthening or weakening.

2.5.2 AMPA receptors (AMPARs)

AMPARs are another class of ionotropic glutamate receptors that mediate most of the fast excitatory synaptic transmission in the brain. They are crucial for both initiation and maintaining of the LTP. Upon the glutamate binding to AMPARs that are predominantly permeable to sodium ions (Na^{+}), these ion channels open and Na^{+} flows into postsynaptic dendrites, resulting in a depolarization of the postsynaptic membrane. This depolarization dissociates magnesium from its binding site within the NMDA receptor channel, thereby allowing the opening of NMDAR upon glutamate binding and resulting in Ca^{2+} influx to the postsynaptic dendrite, which initiates the NMDAR-dependent LTP or LTD [2, 35].

During LTP, the number and conductance of AMPA receptors at the synapse increase, thus enhancing the synaptic strength. In contrast, LTD involves the removal and reduced conductance of AMPA receptors from the synapse, leading to decreased synaptic efficacy.

The endocytosis of AMPA receptors comprising mGluR2 and mGLuR3 subunits also plays a role in the induction of mGluR-dependent LTD in the cerebellar cortex [23].

2.5.3 Calcium signaling and associated pathways

Calcium signaling is central to the processes of LTP and LTD [36, 37]. The entry of Ca^{2+} through NMDARs activates a variety of intracellular signaling cascades that are important for the induction and maintenance of LTP and LTD [2].

For LTP, a brief surge in dendritic spine Ca^{2+} level activates protein kinases, most importantly the Ca^{2+}/calmodulin-dependent protein kinase II (CaMKII), which in turn phosphorylates synaptic proteins, and together with the small GTP-binding protein Rab11a, it promotes the insertion of AMPA receptors into the synapse. The new synaptic AMPARs are stabilized through their transmembrane AMPAR regulatory protein (TARP)-mediated interaction with PDZ domain-containing proteins such as PSD-95 (postsynaptic density 95). CaMKII also phosphorylates AMPA receptors and enhances their single-channel conductance [38, 39]. Hence, the postsynaptic membrane is more prepared for depolarization upon ligand binding to AMPARs and activates NMDA ion channels when they bind to glutamate to allow further Ca^{2+} influx.

For LTD, a prolonged moderate increase in postsynaptic Ca^{2+} level activates protein phosphatases primarily calcineurin and protein phosphatases 1, which dephosphorylate synaptic proteins such as Ser-845 of the AMPAR GluR1 subunit and lead to the internalization and removal of synaptic AMPA receptors, while reducing the probability of opening AMPA receptor channels as well. Thus, the postsynaptic membrane becomes less excitable and the permeability of NMDA ion channels for Ca^{2+} is decreased, which results in a smaller influx of Ca^{2+} into the postsynaptic neuron and ends in the process for LTD.

Calcium signaling is widely involved in other types of synaptic plasticity as well. As mentioned before, a transient accumulation of Ca^{2+} in presynaptic axonal end takes part into the induction of short-term synaptic plasticity.

2.5.4 Protein kinase A (PKA)

PKA phosphorylation of the AMPA receptor subunits GluR4 and GluR1 directly controls the synaptic incorporation of AMPARs into synapses. PKA phosphorylation of GluR4 relieves the retention of AMPAR and drives it into synapse, while PKA phosphorylation of GluR1, together with CaMKII, plays important roles in AMPA receptor incorporation into the synapse [40]. In addition, PKA also exists presynaptically and plays an important role in the mossy fiber LTP, the cAMP-dependent presynaptic form of plasticity. PKA interacts with proteins in the cAMP-bound protein complex including SV2, Rim1, and SNAP25, hence modulating the production of the readily releasable pool of synaptic vesicles and therefore modulating the release of neurotransmitters [41]. PKA is activated by the Ca^{2+}-stimulated adenylyl cyclase.

2.6 Roles in neural circuit function and plasticity

These mechanisms of synaptic plasticity are essential for the dynamic regulation of neural circuits. By strengthening or weakening specific synaptic connections, LTP and LTD enable the brain to store and retrieve information, adapt to new experiences, and maintain homeostasis. Short-term synaptic plasticity influences the information processing function of synapses based on their initial probability of substance release, thus serving as high-pass or low-pass filters and modulating synaptic efficacy continuously on very short time scales [42, 43]. Proper functioning of these processes is vital for emotional responses and cognitive functions such as learning and memory, while their dysregulation can lead to various neurological disorders.

3. Pathological synaptic plasticity: General concepts

3.1 Defining pathological synaptic plasticity

Plasticity is the capacity of our nervous system to generate neural activity based on experience to modify neural circuit function and thereby modify subsequent thoughts, feelings and behavior.

Normal synaptic plasticity is the activity-dependent modification of the strength or efficacy of synaptic transmission at pre-existing synapses [8]. It can act to reorganize the structure and function of neurons and ensure that the brain can adapt to new information, experiences, and environmental changes. Normal synaptic plasticity facilitates learning, memory, and adaptive neural circuit modulation, also allowing the network to remain robust and stable over time [44].

Pathological synaptic plasticity shows the deficits in environmental and experience-mediated modification of synaptic strength and results in the maladaptive changes that impair synaptic function and neural network stability. Pathological plasticity often leads to the excessive strengthening or weakening of synapses, which disrupts the balance of neural circuits and impairs cognitive and motor functions. It disturbs processes including learning and memory, leading to cognitive deficits, behavioral abnormalities, and neurodegeneration.

3.2 Dysregulation in synaptic plasticity mechanisms and disease

Dysregulation in synaptic plasticity mechanisms can lead to several neurological diseases. The precise mechanisms through which this occurs vary by disorders but often involve alterations in key molecular players such as NMDA receptors, AMPA receptors, and calcium signaling pathways.

3.3 Common features of pathological synaptic plasticity across disorders

Despite the diverse etiologies and manifestations of neurological disorders, several common features of pathological synaptic plasticity can be identified across different conditions:

Synaptic imbalance: Many disorders exhibit an imbalance between excitatory and inhibitory synaptic transmission, leading to network instability.

Dysregulated synaptic receptor Function: Alterations in the function or expression of synaptic receptors (e.g., NMDAR and AMPAR) are common in various neurological diseases.

Impaired synaptic homeostasis: The failure to maintain synaptic homeostasis and plasticity results in the progressive loss of synaptic integrity and function.

Abnormal build-up of proteins: The induction and maintenance of synaptic plasticity depend on the normal function of multiple synaptic proteins including postsynaptic density (PSD) and neurotransmitter receptors, as well as the activity of downstream signaling pathways. Mutations in genes encoding proteins affecting synaptic plasticity and the protein misfolding would damage the normal synaptic plasticity.

Understanding these commonalities helps to elucidate the underlying mechanisms of disease and identify potential therapeutic targets to alleviate the effects of pathological synaptic plasticity.

4. Neurological disorders associated with pathological synaptic plasticity

Patients with early-stage neurodegenerative diseases and some other neurological disorders such as epilepsy show significant instabilities in neurological functions, which are clearly not an outcome of sudden changes in the number of neurons. It is more reasonable to consider that the fluctuations are caused by the alternations in the activity of the neural network, in which synapses and synaptic plasticity play crucial roles and their deficits might be compensated temporarily.

4.1 Alzheimer's disease

Alzheimer's disease is an aging-dependent neurodegenerative disorder characterized by a progressive decline in cognitive function. It is closely associated with synaptic dysfunction and loss [45]. In Alzheimer's disease, the synaptic loss seems to be more prominent than the neuronal loss, and the depletion of synapses and synaptic proteins correlates better with cognitive decline than other pathological markers do [46–50]. Synaptic degeneration precedes neuronal death [51]. Functional MRI has shown that individuals with a genetic tendency for Alzheimer's disease displayed a thinner entorhinal cortex even during the childhood [52], and there is a specific loss of dendritic spine heads in the entorhinal cortex that serves as an interface between the hippocampus and neocortical regions and contributes to memory acquisition and retrieval [53]. Studies on post-mortem brain tissues also showed a decrease in the expression of both NMDA and AMPA receptors [54] and their subunits [55–59]. These findings indicate a disruption of synaptic plasticity, which is certainly related to the deficits of cognition in Alzheimer's disease. Moreover, as compared to the general population, patients suffered from Alzheimer's disease showed two to six folds of increase in the incidence of epileptic seizures [60–62], suggesting alterations in the regulation of synaptic activity and a loss of balance of the neural network.

The neuropathology underlying the abnormal plasticity includes the deposits of insoluble amyloid β-peptide (Aβ) in extracellular plaques, which is characteristic for Alzheimer's disease. There are persistent alterations in plasticity mechanisms in animal models of amyloidopathy, in particular the impairment of LTP and enhancement of LTD [63–65]. Mice over-expressing human amyloid precursor protein with mutations linked to familial Alzheimer's disease showed synaptic alterations and deficits in LTP in hippocampus and prefrontal cortex [66, 67]. Interestingly, injection of the 42 amino acid form of amyloid-β (Aβ42) at a very low concentration (picomolar level) into mouse hippocampus enhanced synaptic plasticity and memory, whereas the application of Aβ42 at a higher concentration (nanomolar level) impaired synaptic plasticity and memory [68]. These data suggest that Aβ at physiological concentration has a beneficial effect on synaptic plasticity, while the excess of Aβ becomes toxic and causes damage to normal synaptic plasticity. One common phenotype of all animal models of amyloidopathy is the reduction of gamma (γ) oscillation (in human, frequency 25–140 Hz, the 40 Hz point is of particular interest) and slowing of theta (θ) oscillation [69]. These animal models showed increased susceptibility to seizure, which is in agreement with the findings in Alzheimer patients.

Another characteristic neuropathological change of the Alzheimer's disease is the presence of aggregated tau protein. Physiological tau is mostly expressed in the axons and mainly serves as a microtubule stabilizer. Moreover, tau phosphorylation is required for hippocampal LTD, and phosphorylated tau helps to promote endocytosis and internalization of synaptic AMPAR [70]. In Alzheimer subjects, hyperphosphorylated tau dissociates from microtubules and forms neurofibrilliary tangles that is detectable in the brain 2 to 5 years before the symptoms appear. The tau pathology is considered to better reflect cognition changes [71, 72]. Synapse is particularly vulnerable to tau-mediated disruption. Hyperphosphorylated tau is preferentially located at synapses, while mouse models either expressing specific tau isoforms [73–75] or over-expressing disease associated tau mutations exhibited loss of synapses [76]. It has been shown that tau pathology altered synaptic plasticity. Intracellular infusion of tau into neurons of mouse brain slices markedly impair the induction of LTP [77], while extracellular application of tau oligomers to mouse brain slices or directly into mouse brains also impaired LTP [78, 79]. Chronic mouse models of tauopathy have shown alterations in both long-term and short-term plasticity as well [80, 81].

In addition, there seems to be a mechanistic link between pathological Aβ and tau [82]. Aβ oligomers enhance the probability of presynaptic glutamate release, which in turn increases the extrasynaptic NMDAR activation, thus promoting the induction of NMDAR-dependent LTD. The consequent excessive activation of LTD-associated kinases results in hyperphosphorylation of tau at non-physiological residues. The hyperphosphorylated tau then causes further damage to the synaptic plasticity in brains with Alzheimer's disease.

4.2 Parkinson's disease

Parkinson's disease is a chronic neurodegenerative disorder that causes problems with movement, mental health, sleep, pain and other health issues. The motor symptoms usually emerge first and include bradykinesia, tremor, rigidity, and imbalance. The most characteristic pathophysiological change of Parkinson's disease is the progressive loss of dopaminergic neurons in substantia nigra *pars compacta* (SNc) [83, 84], which results in disrupted basal ganglia loop that is involved in motor control. The basal ganglia (BG) are a collection of subcortical structures consisting striatum (caudate, putamen and nucleus accumbens), globus pallidus (GP), subthalamic nucleus (STN) and substantia nigra (SN). These structures are interconnected and connected to cerebral cortex and thalamus and give rise to the direct, indirect, and hyperdirect pathways that modulate locomotion. The striatum is the largest of the basal ganglia nuclei and is one of the two recipients receiving topographically organized excitatory inputs from cerebral cortex and thalamus. Most of the neurons in striatum are GABAergic spiny projecting neurons (SPNs). They can be defined into two types of SPNs based on their involvements in the direct or indirect pathways: the direct pathway SPNs (dSPNs) that project directly to internal GP (GPi)/substantia nigra *pars reticulata* (SNr) – the major output center of BG that transmit processed information to downstream motor regions; and the indirect pathway SPNs (iSPNs) that project to external GP (GPe) where the information was further processed and then sent to GPi/SNr indirectly [85, 86]. Briefly, the direct pathway serves as the movement initiator, and the information flow in direct pathway can be depicted as: *cortex → striatum → GPi/SNr → thalamus → motor cortex*. On the contrary, the indirect pathway serves as the movement terminator; the information flow can be depicted as: *cortex → striatum → GPe → STN → GPi/SNr → thalamus → motor cortex* (**Figure 1A**). The hyperdirect pathway bypasses striatum, conveys signals from cortex directly to subthalamus, and modulates baseline activities; it can be depicted as *cortex → STN → GPi/SNr → thalamus → cortex* (**Figure 1B**). Dopaminergic transmission regulates the direct and indirect pathway activities as well as synaptic plasticity via D1 and D2 receptors [87]. The striatal dSPNs express D1 receptors whose activation increases somatodendritic excitability, enhances glutamatergic transmission, and facilitates LTP; whereas the iSPNs express D2 receptors whose activation decreases intrinsic excitability, attenuates glutamatergic transmission, and promotes LTD [88, 89].

Loss of dopaminergic neurons in SNc decreases the dopamine level in BG and causes an activity imbalance between the direct and indirect pathways. In rat and mouse models of Parkinson's disease, the activation of striatal iSPNs and the inhibition of dSPNs were observed [90, 91]. In addition, the firing rate of dSPNs upon cortical stimulation reduced after partial nigrostriatal DA depletion, whereas no changes were seen in iSPNs, suggesting a functional disconnection of dSPNs from motor cortex, and this disconnection occurred even in mice without symptoms. Moreover, in symptomatic mice, iSPNs fired not only significantly more but also earlier than dSPNs, indicating that both the strength and timing of the direct and indirect pathways were altered in response to partial nigrostriatal DA depletion [92]. Furthermore, it has been noticed that dopaminergic depletion selectively decreased the spontaneous activities of those corticostriatal neurons preferentially synapsed on dSPNs [90] and selectively decreased synaptic strength of thalamic inputs to dSPNs as well [93]. Thus, degeneration of SNc dopaminergic neurons causes a cascade of imbalances in the entire basal ganglia-thalamo-cortical circuit, and the disruption in function occurs prior to the onset of motor symptoms.

Adaptive changes at the synaptic level following dopaminergic deficiency underlie the circuitry disruption. In parkinsonian D1-receptor-KO mice, the spine density decreases in both dSPNs and iSPNs, and this spine loss in iSPNs, but not dSPNs, can be reversed by chronic levodopa administration [94]. Therefore, dopamine and its receptors are essential for the maintenance of spine plasticity at least in dSPNs, and the

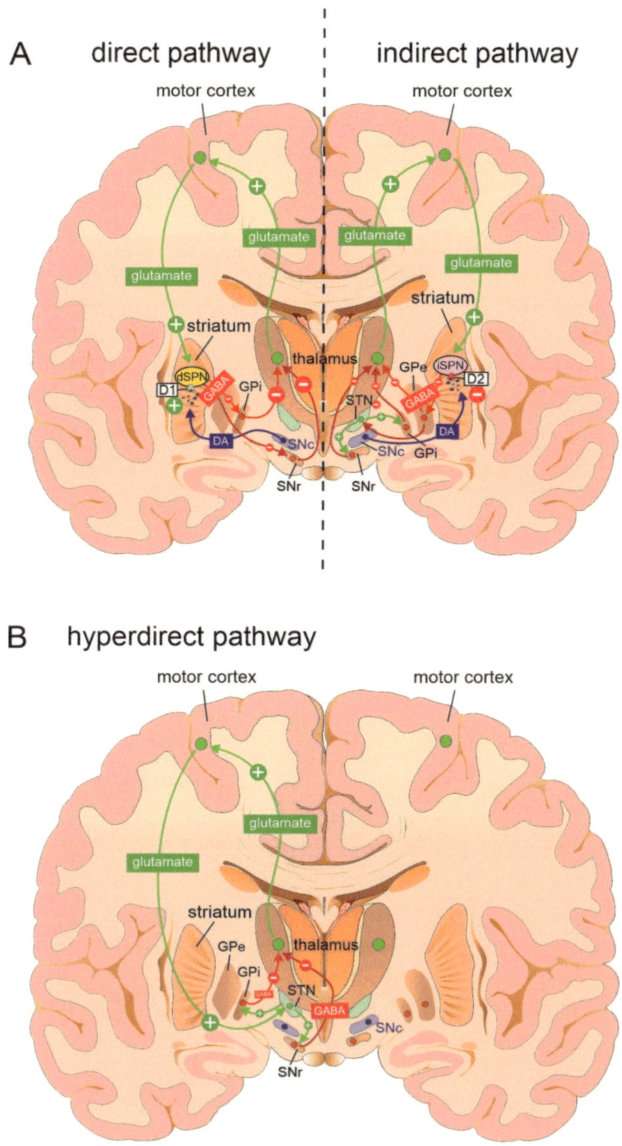

Figure 1.
Diagram of three basal ganglia pathways that are engaged in the control of movement. Green dots represent the excitatory glutamatergic neurons; red dots represent the inhibitory GABAergic neurons; blue dots represent the dopaminergic neurons. The axonal projections are shown by lines and arrows; green lines and "+" indicate excitatory effects; and red lines and "-" indicate inhibitory effects. (A) Left side: the major components and connections of the direct pathway. The excitatory glutamatergic pyramidal neurons (green dots) in the cortex project to the striatum and stimulate the inhibitory GABAergic spiny projecting neurons (SPNs) in striatum. In addition, the SPNs involved in the direct pathways (dSPNs) express dopaminergic D1 receptors and are also activated by dopamine released from dopaminergic inputs originated in the substantia nigra pars compacta (SNc). These dSPNs project to internal globus pallidas (GPi) and substantia nigra pars reticulata (SNr), from where the inhibitory GABAergic neurons (red dots) further send out axons to thalamus. The excitatory glutamatergic thalamic neurons then send projections back to motor cortex. Right side: the major components and connections of the indirect pathway. The excitatory glutamatergic pyramidal neurons (green dots) in the cortex project to the striatum to activate the inhibitory GABAergic SPNs in striatum, whereas the SPNs involved in the indirect pathways (iSPNs) express dopaminergic D2 receptors and are inhibited by dopamine released from dopaminergic neurons in SNc. These iSPNs project to external globus pallidas (GPe), the inhibitory GABAergic in GPe then project to GPi and SNr, from where the inhibitory GABAergic neurons (red dots) further send projections to thalamus. Finally, the excitatory glutamatergic thalamic neurons project back to the motor cortex.

(B) The major components and connections of the hyperdirect pathway. The excitatory glutamatergic pyramidal neurons (green dots) in the cortex send projections that bypass striatum and reach the subthalamic nucleus (STN). Then, the excitatory glutamatergic neurons in STN also send projections to GPi and SNr, same as in the other two pathways, thalamus receives inputs from GPi and SNr, and the excitatory glutamatergic thalamic neurons project back to motor cortex. Abbreviations: dSPNs, direct pathway spiny projecting neurons; iSPNs, indirect pathway spiny projecting neurons; GPe, external globus pallidas; GPi, internal globus pallidas; SNc, substantia nigra pars compacta; SNr, substantia nigra pars reticulata; SPNs, spiny projecting neurons in striatum; STN, subthalamic nucleus.

damage cannot be rescued afterwards. In addition to D1 or D2 receptors, both dSPNs and iSPNs also express AMPAR, NMDAR, and metabolic glutamatergic receptors that mediate synaptic transmission and LTP/LTD. The iSPNs also express adenosine A2a receptor, which couples to the same second messenger cascades as D1 receptors do [95]. Antagonizing these A2a receptors or blocking MNDA receptors disrupted the induction of LTP in iSPNs. Conversely, activation of the A2a receptor in combination with D2 receptor blockage led to the induction of LTP. In case of dSPNs, the activation of NMDA and D1 receptors induced LTP, whereas activation of musacarinic M4 receptor and mGluR5 induced LTD [96]. These data demonstrate that dopamine, in concert with glutamate, adenosine and acetylcholine, induces bidirectional plasticity at glutamatergic synapses formed on striatal SPNs. This bidirectional regulatory balance was absent in Parkinsonian models. In the hypo-dopaminergic state, plasticity at glutamatergic synapses is still present, but it has lost its bidirectionality. Therefore, without dopamine, no D1 activation on dSPNs and they lose LTP, only exhibit LTD; while no D2 activation on iSPNs and they lose LTD, only exhibit LTP [96, 97]. This DA-deficiency-induced unidirectional synaptic plasticity at corticostriatal synapses plays a critical role in the disruption of the balance between activities of dSPNs and iSPNs, thus disturbing the normal motor control and motor learning [98]. eCB-LTD also exists on SPNs and is one of the best-characterized forms of corticostriatal synaptic plasticity [2]. eCB-LTD is primarily restricted to the iSPNs and mediates the depression of synapses in the indirect pathway. This eCB-LTD-mediated depression plays a critical role in motor control. It is absent in Parkinson's disease models, but can be rescued by activation of D2 receptor or inhibition of endocannabinoid degradation [99].

One of the key pathological hallmarks of Parkinson's disease is the presence of Lewy bodies in neurons of Parkinsonian brains. Alpha-synuclein (α-Syn) is thought to be primarily responsible for Lewy body aggregation [100, 101]. Genome-wide association studies also link α-Syn to sporadic forms of Parkinson's disease [102]. In a triple $\alpha/\beta/\gamma$-synuclein-knockout mouse model, eCB-LTD is abolished, but no changes in the basal corticostriatal synaptic transmission, and presynaptic CB1 receptors are not affected either. The abolished eCB-LTD is caused by impaired endocannabinoid release as postsynaptic release of endocannabinoid requires α-Syn [103]. Hence, α-Syn dysfunction underlies the disruption of eCB-LTD in Parkinson's disease.

4.3 Schizophrenia

Schizophrenia is a major psychiatric disorder characterized by disturbances in perception, attention, volition, inferential thinking, speech, and emotion. The disturbance in cognition is considered as a core feature of schizophrenia [104]. One common cognitive deficit in schizophrenic subjects is the impaired working memory, which is associated to prominent disturbances in the circuitry of dorsolateral prefrontal cortex (DLPFC). There is a decrease in excitatory inputs to DLPFC deep layer III pyramidal neurons [105–107], consequently reducing excitatory outputs from these glutamatergic neurons to the GABAergic interneurons, in particular the parvalbumin (PV)-containing chandelier neurons in DLPFC. This weakens the GABAergic inhibitory transmission as the expression of the 67-kDa isoform of glutamic acid decarboxylase (GAD_{67}), an enzyme that regulates GABA synthesis, depends on the amount of excitatory activity these neurons received [108]. The decreased GABAergic transmission in turn causes disinhibition of pyramidal neurons and an excess of glutamate at the non-NMDA receptors, hence disrupting the cortical circuit function [109]. The disruption of the DLPFC circuitry contributes to the working memory dysfunction in schizophrenic subjects. Indeed, it was supported by a clinical trial showing that the glutamatergic autoreceptor agonist that inhibits the presynaptic glutamate release has antipsychotic effects [110]. Thus, the disturbance of normal brain microcircuits is one of the major neuropathological features of schizophrenia and is also considered as a common underlying feature in neuropsychiatric diseases [111].

Synapses are functional units of neural circuits, and synaptic plasticity controls the information flow between neurons in the network. In schizophrenia, the disruption of synaptic function includes altered glutamate and GABA transmission, altered expression of synaptic molecules, and the loss of dendritic spines. One fundamental alteration in schizophrenia is the NMDAR hypofunction, which has been supported by both pharmacological and gene expression evidences. Administration of low-dose NMDAR antagonists such as phencyclidine or ketamine to normal subjects induced a broad range of schizophrenic symptoms including both positive and negative symptoms and the cognitive impairments [112–114]. Moreover, the observation that most of the patients suffered from the NMDAR-antibody encephalitis (the encephalitis associated with antibodies against the NMDA receptor) developed schizophrenic symptoms further confirmed the neuropathological role of NMDAR deficiency in schizophrenia [115, 116]. Studies on post-mortem samples have also shown significant decreases in the mRNA expression levels of NMDAR subunits GluN1 and GluN2C in the prefrontal cortex of schizophrenic subjects [117, 118], and there were striking decreases in postsynaptic NMDAR-mediated signaling in DLPFC [119]. Genetic variation in the subunit of calcineurin, which is thought to play an important role in NMDAR-dependent LTD, has been associated with schizophrenia [120], while knocking out the calcineurin subunit encoding gene specifically in mouse forebrain created working memory deficiency and other schizophrenia-like deficits [121]. Antipsychotics such as lithium, valproate, and lamotrigine have significant effects on the phosphorylation of AMPAR subunits and affect their surface expression [122–124]. Therefore, NMDAR hypofunction and most likely the associated impairment of synaptic plasticity is one of the major pathological changes in schizophrenia.

Accumulating evidence has suggested that alterations in short-term synaptic plasticity might play a dominant role in the synaptic pathology of schizophrenia [111]. Characteristic cognitive deficits in schizophrenia including the impaired working memory suggest a disturbance in the moment-to-moment information processing carried out by the neural circuits [125, 126]. Numerous schizophrenia candidate risk genes and genetic mutations have been identified, and the variants are significant. However, mouse models based upon the most relevant and highly penetrant risk variants have shown more consistent alterations in short-term synaptic plasticity, which strongly implicates a presynaptic site of dysfunction [127, 128]. For example, human subjects with hypomorphic mutations in the *PRODH* (proline dehydrogenase 1) gene showed higher incidence of schizophrenia and schizoaffective disorder, while electrophysiological studies of the *PRODH*-knockdown mice suggested that PRODH (a mitochondrial protein that catalyzes the first step in proline degradation) deficiency altered the synaptic plasticity via increasing the initial probability of presynaptic neurotransmitter release and an inability of LTP induction that would further increase the initial probability of presynaptic neurotransmitter release [129]. Similarly but via different mechanisms, deficiency of another two schizophrenia risk genes *RGS4* (regulator of G-protein signaling) and *Dtnbp1* (dysbindin) were shown to reduce the probability of presynaptic neurotransmitter release and cause alterations in short-term plasticity in neural circuits (reviewed in [111]). In addition, the *DISC1* (disrupted in schizophrenia 1) gene-encoded DISC1 scaffold protein is involved in neurite outgrowth and cortical development and probably plays a significant role in regulating presynaptic short-term plasticity mechanisms. The disruption of the *DISC1* gene is associated with familial psychoses including schizophrenia [130, 131]. It was found recently that intracellular DISC1 affects the metalloproteinases ADAMTS-4 protein, which in turn is exported and affects the processing of extracellular Reelin and regulates its activity in the perinatal cerebral cortex [132].

Reelin is one of the components of the extracellular matrix (ECM) that regulates neuronal migration and positioning in developing neocortex and cerebellar cortex, while postnatally contributing to synaptic plasticity [133]. Growing evidence has pointed to ECM abnormalities as part of the core pathophysiology of schizophrenia [134]. In addition to pre- and postsynaptic terminals, the concept of "tetrapartite synapse" also includes astroglial processes and synaptic/perisynaptic ECM complexes as a whole functional unit [135]. Astrocytes actively control the synaptic transmission via secretion of various molecules such as D-serine, which acts as a co-agonist for NMDARs [136]. ECM forms a mesh mainly on PV-positive interneurons, and its remodeling influences plasticity processes [137]. Human genetic and post-mortem studies show genetic susceptibilities for genes encoding several important ECM molecules including chondroitin sulfate proteoglycans (CSPGs), Reelin, integrins, and remodeling enzymes like matrix metalloproteases (MMPs). Altered expression of these ECM components in various brain areas were found in schizophrenia subjects, and their disruption in animal models induced abnormalities observed in schizophrenia. Reelin, secreted by a subgroup of interneurons, enhances LTP via regulating the composition of NMDAR and increasing the number of postsynatptic AMPARs [138, 139]. The interaction between integrin and other ECM components such as Reelin regulates synaptic plasticity through regulating the AMPAR internalization and surface mobility of NMDAR subunits [140, 141]. Perineuronal net (PNN) is a specific form of highly organized CSPGs that tightly surround synaptic contacts on the soma, dendrites, and axon initial segments. PNNs are predominantly present on the PV-positive interneurons and play a key role in synaptic regulation, especially the glutamatergic synapses [134]. PNNs hinder the lateral diffusion of AMPA receptors between synaptic and extrasynaptic compartments and modulate synaptic plasticity [142], while mice lacking key PNN component tenascin-R showed marked decrease in LTP [143]. Thus, PNN abnormalities may alter the efficacy of synapses and transmitter release associated with schizophrenia [144, 145]. Moreover, it has been found that there is an obvious decrease in dendritic spines in prefrontal and auditory cortices and hippocampus in schizophrenic subjects. The ECM proteins and their surface receptors, as well as remodeling ECM enzymes such as MMP-9, are involved in regulating dendritic spine plasticity in adulthood, and thus the ECM aberration might contribute to the loss of dendritic spines in schizophrenia [146].

4.4 Autism spectrum disorders (ASD)

Autism spectrum disorder is a heterogeneous neurodevelopmental disease characterized by deficits in communication skills (verbal and non-verbal) and repetitive patterns of behavior, speech, or activities. Similar to schizophrenia, autism is also a disease of abnormal synaptic plasticity and connectivity. Studies on valproic acid rat model of autism and functional imaging studies in autism indicated hyper-connectivity and hyper-plasticity in local microcircuitry and short-range connections [147–153], but a decreased connectivity in long-range connections between different brain regions [154]. Taken together, the circuitry [147] in autism is mainly the hyper-functioning and hyper-plasticity of local neural microcircuits, which is different from the hypofunction and hypoplasticity of microcircuits observed in schizophrenia. This microcircuit pathology matches core cognitive consequences of autism including *hyper-perception, hyper-attention, hyper-memory, and hyper-emotionality*. Comprehensive analyses of functional neuroimaging and phenotypic data obtained from subjects with autism together with computational modeling found alterations in subcortical (in particular thalamic) drive into cortical microcircuits, together with alterations in excitation/inhibition [155]. Genetic studies and large patient population genome analyses have identified a number of risk genes that are known to regulate synaptic function and plasticity (reviewed in [111]), and mouse models based on these risk genes have shown both short-term and long-term synaptic plasticity alterations [156].

The most significant genetic findings relevant to ASD are the single-gene mutations identified in fragile X syndrome [157, 158], Rett's syndrome [159], and Phelan-McDermid syndrome [160].

Fragile X syndrome (FXS) is the most common monogenetic neurodevelopmental disorder associated with ASD. The affected gene *FMR1* (fragile X messenger ribonucleoprotein 1) is located on chromosome X. Expansions of CGG repeat in most cases or in rare cases point mutations/deletions in the *FMR1* gene result in absent or markedly decrease of its production of the FMRP (fragile X mental retardation protein), which is an RNA-binding protein enriched in neurons (both in soma and dendrites) and serves as a negative regulator of the translation of many mRNAs [161]. This function of FMRP has been confirmed by both *in vivo* and *in vitro* studies on *Fmr1*-null mice showing that there was an increase in basal protein synthesis in hippocampal areas of these mice. This enhanced translation could be restored to the normal level by inhibiting mGluR5 or ERK1/2 [162, 163], which is in agreement with the finding that mGluR-dependent LTD is exaggerated in the hippocampus of *Fmr1*-knockout mice [164]. It has been discovered that FMRP is synthesized at synapses in response to application of glutamate or mGluR agonists. Both mGluR1 and mGluR5 are located at synapse and seem to be part of the protein translation machinery for the synthesis of synaptic proteins including FMRP in response to synaptic stimulation, and the increase in FMRP after stimulation is fast [165]. Thus, the synaptic activity modulates the level of synaptic FMRP, which in turn regulates synaptic function and plasticity through limiting the rapid translation at synapse in response to synaptic stimulation. FMRP dysfunction leads to excessive protein synthesis observed in FXS and caused altered synaptic plasticity [166]. Multiple pathways regulated by FMRP are found to be dysfunctional in ASD patients who do not have FXS [167].

Another monogenetic neurodevelopmental disorder associated with ASD is the Rett syndrome. The affected gene *MECP2* is also located on chromosome X [159]. Mutations in *MECP2* can result in a wide range of symptoms observed in almost all neuropsychiatric disorders including autism, seizures, Parkinsonism, schizophrenia, bipolar disorder, and so on and causes up to 97% of classic Rett syndrome [168, 169]. The protein encoded by *MECP2* is MeCP2, a nuclear protein binds to methylated cytosines [170] and interacts with histone deacetylase-containing complexes to suppress transcription [171, 172]. On the contrary, MeCP2 also binds to promoters of *BDNF* (brain-derived neurotrophic factor gene) and several other neuronal genes and activates their transcription [173–176]. MeCP2 is abundant in neurons [177] and is also expressed in glia with a lower expression level [178–180]. The *Mecp2*-null mouse model developed features of Rett syndrome and showed shrinked PSD, impaired LTP and LTD in hippocampal CA1 region [181, 182], whereas overexpressed *Mecp2* in mice to double the MeCP2 level enhanced LTP in hippocampus and enhanced motor and contextual learning [183]. These data suggest that the alterations in excitatory synaptic plasticity are underlying the cognitive and functional deficits of this disorder. Moreover, deficit of MeCP2 in glia also contributes to the alteration of synaptic plasticity since glia lacking MeCP2 failed to support dendritic morphology of neurons [178, 184].

In addition to aberrations of proteins regulating transcription and translation, deficits of a set of proteins involved in synaptic scaffolding and structure also contribute to the neuropathology of autism. One of them is related to the Phelan-McDermid syndrome (PMS). PMS, also called *22q13* deletion syndrome, is a microdeletion syndrome of chromosome *22q13* characterized by severe neonatal hypotonia, some dysmorphic features, developmental and speech delay, and seizures. *SHANK3* has been identified as the gene responsible for many neurological phenotypes of PMS [160, 185–187]. Mutations in *SHANK3* were found in patients with autism [188, 189]. *SHANK3* is preferentially expressed in the cerebral cortex, hippocampus, and cerebellum and encodes a scaffold protein involved in the PSD of excitatory synapses [160]. Shank1, 2, 3 proteins are components of the PSD and interact with and stabilize the PDS-95/SAPAP/Shank/Homer complexes. Shank proteins also recruit IP3 and F-actin to synapse to enlarge the dendritic spine heads and stabilize them (reviewed in [168]). Shank3 regulates the genesis and structural organization of dendritic spines via interactions with the glutamate receptor complex. It recruits many key functional elements to the PSD and synapse, including components of AMPARs, mGluRs and NMDARs [190]. *Shank3*$^{+/-}$ mice lacking the long isoform showed reduced basal AMPAR-mediated synaptic transmission and impaired LTD [191]. Moreover, Shank3 also binds indirectly to neuroligins, a family of neuronal cell surface proteins. At synapses, some neuroligins act as splice site-specific ligands for the cell surface receptors neurexins to form the Ca^{2+}-dependent neurexin-neuroligin complexes, which is required for efficient neurotransmission. It has been discovered that Shank3 signals to presynaptic boutons through the Neurexin-Neuroligin trans-synaptic signaling complex and regulates the probability of presynaptic neurotransmitter release. Therefore, Shank3 not only regulates AMPAR- and NMDAR-mediated synaptic transmission at the postsynaptic level by controlling the number of these receptors but also simultaneously regulates the neurotransmitter release at the presynaptic level via its interaction with the neurexin-neuroligin complex, hence coordinating both pre- and postsynaptic activity and playing an important regulatory role in synaptic plasticity [192]. Mutations in genes encoding neurexin-1 and 2 have been consistently observed in subjects with autism [193–196], while mutations in genes encoding neuroligin-3 and 4 were also identified [197, 198]. Loss of neuroligin-3 in mice causes some features that are typically seen in ASD patients [199, 200]. A deletion of a neuroligin-4 ortholog in mice caused impaired social interactions and decreased ultrasonic vocalization [201]. Taken together, the synaptic scaffold protein Shank3 regulates postsynaptic transmission and at the same time modulates presynaptic function together with the synaptic neurexin-neuroligin complex. Dysfunction of these proteins impaired synaptic plasticity and contributes to the pathogenesis of autism.

4.5 Epilepsy

Epilepsy is a result of episodic abnormal, excessive, and synchronous discharges in cerebral neural networks. It is characterized by recurrent, unprovoked epileptic seizures and might lead to cognitive decline, temporary neurological dysfunction, brain damage, and other severe consequences such as accidental injury. Neuronal death, synaptic reorganization, and changes in receptor expression have all been implicated in the epileptogenesis.

Human mesial temporal lobe epilepsy (MTLE) is the most common type of intractable partial-onset epilepsy. Most MTLE patients dramatically improved after anterior temporal lobectomy, in which parts of hippocampus, amygdala, and the adjacent temporal cortex were removed, suggesting that these areas are involved in the mechanism underlying the development of MTLE [202]. Most patients have seizure onset within the hippocampal formation [203], and several neuropathological abnormalities were observed. There are neuronal loss and gliosis in hippocampus [203, 204], while the more characteristic change is the sprouting and reorganization of mossy fibers in DG during the latent period that might explain the hippocampal hyperexcitability in patients [205]. The loss of hilar neurons precedes the seizure in rats and is considered to trigger the mossy fiber sprouting [206]. Mossy fibers are axons of DG glutamatergic granule cells, and they normally project to CA3 region. During the epileptogenic process, these fibers sprout recurrent branches and projects back to the inner third of the DG molecular layer to form monosynaptic excitatory connections with other granule cells, thus setting up local excitatory cirucuits, enhancing the granule cell excitability, and inducing cellular hyperexcitability [207, 208]. Moreover, CA1 pyramidal neurons also generate recurrent excitatory collaterals in the CA1 region and cause a hyperexcitability similar to that in DG [202]. Therefore, the synaptic reorganization and sprouting during the genesis of epilepsy and the newly formed neural circuits drive the hippocampal hyperexcitability.

Furthermore, alterations of synaptic receptors change the synaptic property and contribute to the hippocampal hyperexcitability [209]. NMDARs normally do not contribute to the initiation of synaptic potentials but become actively involved in synaptic transmission in kindled hippocampus [210]. mRNA expression levels and patterns of various NMDAR, AMPAR, $GABA_A$, and kainate receptor subunits were altered in kindled hippocampus [211–216], while kindling induced fast and long-lasting posttranslational modifications of NMDAR, enhancing excitability such as phosphorylation of subunits, leading to altered receptor functions including prolonged open time, burst, and duration of NMDA channels as well as reduced channel blocking effect by magnesium [217–219]. In addition, the increased neuronal activity associated with seizure accelerated the constitutive internalization of $GABA_A$ receptors [220], and GABA receptors on dental granule cells became less sensitive to diazepam and Zn^{2+} in the progress of status epilepticus [221, 222], thus diminishing the inhibitory power in neural circuits. An increase in number of functional NMDA receptors per synapse was also observed [223]. In addition, the epileptic discharges are initiated and synchronized by recurrent excitatory collateral connections primarily involving AMPA receptors, whereas the activity of NMDAR is involved in prolonging the duration and reducing the latency of each epileptiform discharge [224–226].

The synaptic rearrangements in hippocampus such as synaptic reorganization and mossy fiber sprouting require a permissive extracellular environment. Therefore, ECM alternations are also involved in neuropathology of epilepsy. Enzymatic digestion of PNNs lower the threshold for seizure induction [227], while PNNs were significantly decreased around PV-positive interneurons after the induction of experimental epilepsy [228]. In general, during development, ECM of the central nervous system transforms from an environment that is conductive to neural plasticity to the one in which synapse formation is restricted toward maturation. PNN plays a role in synaptic stability during adulthood. Changes in PNN were observed in several animal models of epilepsy (reviewed in [229]). For example, neurocan is one of the predominant CSPGs in developing hippocampus and is expressed around the developing mossy fiber tract serving as a barrier for directing mossy fiber extension [230, 231]. Normally, there is very little neurocan expression in adults. However, in Ihara's spontaneous epileptic rats, there is a reappearance of neurocan in the outer molecular layer and hilus at 3 to 8 months of age, which might contribute to mossy fiber sprouting and new synapse formation in DG [232–234]. Kainic acid-induced convulsions also induce prolonged changes in neurocan and phosphacan similar to those in the developing rat brain and suggest a role of these CSPGs in the remodeling of neural networks related to the establishment or enhancement of epileptogenesis [235]. Heterozygous mutations in *RELN*, the gene encoding another ECM protein Reelin, are responsible for about 20% of the autosomal dominant lateral temporal epilepsy that is clinically characterized by focal seizures with auditory symptoms and/or aphasia. The mutant Reelin was not properly secreted into ECM and was degraded by the autophagy pathway [236]. As mentioned before in the "schizophrenia session", Reelin regulates synaptic plasticity, and thus the consequent disruption of synaptic plasticity caused by Reelin deficiency is involved in the pathogenesis of epilepsy.

Moreover, autophagy and the ubiquitin proteasome system are the two major cell-clearing systems that are deeply involved in mechanisms driving synaptic plasticity such as LTP and LTD. The inhibition of either 26S proteasome or autophagy in experimental models produces profound alterations in neurotransmitter release and the expression of neurotransmitter receptors. There is strong correlation between the mTOR (mammalian target of rapamycin)-dependent autophagy and multiple seizure models and epilepsy. mTOR plays multiple roles in brain development, neuronal excitability, and plasticity, as well as inflammation and immunity. mTOR hyperactivation leads to epileptogenesis in human samples and mouse models, whereas inhibition of mTOR prevents the development of epilepsy and underlying neuronal alterations. Abnormal autophagy pathway might cause alterations in a variety of cell functions including synaptic plasticity and contribute to epileptogenesis [237–239].

On the other hand, it has been shown that LTP is markedly reduced at the epileptic focus (hippocampus) in humans with temporal lobe epilepsy, and impaired synaptic plasticity may contribute to deficient declarative memory in human temporal lobe epilepsy [240]. In animal models, kindling or electrically induced seizures suppress or block LTP and impair learning and memory [241–243]. Astrocytes modulate short- and long-term synaptic plasticity and neuronal excitability via Ca^{2+}-dependent neurotransmitter release from astrocytes [244–246]. It was then found that glutamatergic CA3-CA1 synapses from kindled rats exhibit an impaired LTP, which is accompanied by an increased probability of neurotransmitter release and an abnormal pattern of astroglial Ca^{2+}-dependent transients. Blocking of purinergic P2Y1 receptors with specific antagonist reversed the alterations in LTP and probability of neurotransmitter release, suggesting that astrocytes might take part in the mechanisms that deteriorate synaptic plasticity and caused the cognitive decline in epileptic patients [247].

5. Current and emerging therapeutic strategies

The long-term progress of neurodegenerative disorders allows the brain to engage compensatory mechanisms. Optimizing the plasticity of remaining neural networks would help patients to function as well as possible within the limits of leftover neural structures. There are various therapeutic strategies aiming at modulating synaptic plasticity including pharmacological and non-pharmacological interventions, gene therapy and CRISPR-based approaches, and lifestyle and behavioral interventions.

5.1 Pharmacological interventions

Both NMDA and AMPA receptors are key players in synaptic plasticity; their dysfunction is implicated in various neurological disorders. Modulating NMDA and AMPA receptor activities is a promising therapeutic approach.

NMDAR antagonists potentially have a wide range of therapeutic applications, which include Alzheimer's disease, Parkinson's disease, schizophrenia, and epilepsy. Memantine is an uncompetitive NMDAR antagonist having neuroprotective activity at the therapeutic dose and lacking negative effects typically observed with several different NMDAR antagonists. It attenuated disruption of neuronal plasticity produced by tonic over stimulation of NMDAR *in vitro* and was effective in treating Parkinson's disease [248]. Moreover, it is clinically well tolerated, and the administration of memantine in combination with cholinesterase inhibitors has shown reliable efficacy in improving cognition [249, 250]. The partial NMDAR agonist D-Cycloserine binds to the D-serine/glycine binding site of the NMDAR and augments LTP, and it also positively modulates LTD, thus enhancing memory consolidation [251]. Preliminary trials in patients with schizophrenia suggest that DCS may produce persistent improvement of negative symptoms and enhance learning when combined with cognitive behavioral therapy for delusions or with cognitive remediation [252].

Ampakines bind to a site on the AMPA receptor but have no agonist or antagonist effects; instead, they keep the AMPA ion channel open for longer period and prolong the current flow, hence enhancing synaptic responses. They also lower the induction threshold and increase the magnitude of LTP, thus helping learning. Ampakines improve synaptic plasticity as well and protect neurons against neurotoxic insults by increasing concentrations of BDNF in the brain. They were found effective in correcting behaviors in various animal models of schizophrenia [253–255]. However, their therapeutic potential has since declined due to inconsistent results in clinical trials.

BDNF is a brain-derived neurotrophic factor that is abundant in the brain and is involved in all levels of neuroplasticity including synaptic plasticity [256] and is used as a marker of plasticity in clinical trials [257]. Synaptic dysfunction of the nucleus tractus solitarius of *Mecp2*-null mice was found to be accompanied by decreased BDNF, while exogenous BDNF administration to the brain stem preparation rescued the synaptic defects [258]. The increase in BDNF level seems to be a ubiquitous consequence of many established and effective psychiatric treatments. For example, memantine, ampakines, ketamine, and lithium treatments all elevate BDNF levels

[259–262], and other therapies such as the non-invasive brain stimulation (NIBS) techniques also upregulate BDNF levels [263]. BDNF exerts its function via tropomyosin receptor kinase B (TrkB) and the downstream signaling pathways such as the MAPK/ERK and Ras-PI3K-Akt pathways that are essential for neurogenesis, neurite outgrowth, and promoting neuronal survival [264]. Therefore, BDNF is a novel therapeutic focus for neurodegenerative disorders.

5.2 Non-pharmacological interventions

Transcranial magnetic stimulation (TMS) is a non-invasive technique that uses magnetic fields to stimulate neural activity. It is used to treat various psychiatric and neurological conditions. One advantage of this therapy is its ability to induce plasticity even long after the treatment. Basically, high-frequency TMS elicits LTP; low-frequency TMS elicits LTD [265]. Theta-burst stimulation (TBS) is a new form of repetitive TMS; intermittent TBS mimics the endogenous brain theta rythms, alters gamma oscillations that are necessary for neocortical cognitive functions, and improves working memory performance [266]. TMS applied to DLPFC of patients with depression normalized the cortical activity that was often hypoactive without treatments and improved mood [267, 268]. Repetitive TMS emulates aspects of activity-dependent plasticity [269]. Repetitive TMS applied to Wernicke's area (left temporoparietal region) induced LTD and alleviated auditory/verbal hallucination in subjects suffered from schizophrenia or schizoaffective disorder [270]. Thus, TMS can normalize aberrant connection and circuits in various neural and psychiatric disorders and show efficacies in improving cognition, mood, and relieve hallucinations.

Gamma oscillations (30–90 Hz) are thought to be important for higher cognitive functions and sensory responses. Optogenetic stimulation might be used to help to rescue the alteration in gamma oscillation, a deficit that has been observed in several neurological and psychiatric disorders. In a mouse model of Alzheimer's disease (5XFAD mice), reduced behaviorally-driven gamma oscillation was seen before the onset of plaque formation or cognitive decline. Optogenetically driving FS-PV-interneurons at gamma (40 Hz), but not other frequencies, reduced levels of amyloid-β (Aβ)1-40 and Aβ1-42 isoforms. Moreover, the 40 Hz stimulation activated microglia toward a phagocytic state and increased the microglial uptake of Aβ [271]. Based on the previous finding that visual stimulation can drive oscillations in the gamma range, the same researchers exposed 5XFAD mice to 40 Hz light flickering for 1 hour and induced gamma oscillation, which in turn activated microglia and reduced Aβ1-40 and Aβ1-42 levels in the visual cortex of pre-depositing mice and mitigated plaque load in aged, depositing mice. In addition, the same 40 Hz visual flicker (7 days of 1 hour treatment) applied to the TauP301S tauopathy mouse model significantly reduced phosphorylated tau serine202 and serine404/threonine403/serine400 levels in the visual cortex. Similarly, the auditory stimulation with a train of tones flickering at 40 Hz improved spatial and recognition memory and reduced amyloid in auditory cortex and hippocampus of 5XFAD mice [272]. Thus, the 40 Hz light-flickering and auditory stimulation, named as gamma entrainment using sensory stimulus (GENUS), could be a potential valuable non-invasive therapeutic approach for treating neurodegenerative disorders like Alzheimer's disease. Similarly, gamma oscillation in patients with schizophrenia is attenuated during various cognitively demanding tasks including attention, memory, and object representation, [273–278], and reduced gamma oscillations at rest and during sensory processing and facial presentation task was observed in autism [279]. GENUS might also be applied as an additional therapy in treating schizophrenia and autism.

5.3 Gene therapy

Gene therapy offers the potential to precisely target and correct genetic mutations that underlie pathological synaptic plasticity. It is carried out *in vitro*, involving the genetic modification of cultured cells and transplanting them into the patient, or *in vivo*, involving the use of vectors to deliver nucleic acids (DNA, RNA, etc.) or genome-modifying components such as CRISPR-Cas to cells/tissues to correct a mutation or to regulate a gene's expression. There are few ongoing clinical trials of gene therapy for Pakinson's disease. For example, *Lrrk2* mutations cause familial Pakinson's disease. Intracerebral injection of antisense oligonucleotides targeting *Lrrk2* in mice reduced fibril-induced α-synuclein inclusions and protected tyrosine hydroxylase-positive neurons. A Phase I clinical trial using *LRRK2* anti-sense oligonucleotides intrathecal injections (NCT03976349) is ongoing to examine the effect of LRRK2 depletion in the brain. Mutations in *GBA1* gene encoding glucocerebrosidase beta 1 cause Gaucher's disease and is a common risk factor for developing Parkinson's disease [280]. An AAV9 vector-based gene therapy designed to deliver a functional *GBA1* gene to the brain to treat Parkinsonic patients is recently studied in two phase I/II clinical trials (NCT04127578) [281].

5.4 Behavioral interventions and physical exercise

Cognitive behavioral therapy (CBT) is a structured, time-limited psychotherapy that aims to change patterns of thinking or behavior that contribute to a person's problems. Distributed prefrontal neural systems underlie perception, cognition, social interactions, emotion regulation, and motivation. There is a high degree of learning-dependent plasticity in the neural circuits. Successful cognitive training might re-establish proper synaptic plasticity and improve the impaired neural systems in neuropsychiatric disorders [282]. The gross thinning of cortices associated with symptom severity and cognition deficits has been found in schizophrenic patients. It has been shown that targeted cognitive training (TCT) improved cognition and reduced cortical thinning in frontal, temporal, parietal, and occipital lobes [283]. Thalamus plays a crucial role in the integration of neuronal signals across cortical and subcortical brain areas, and disrupted thalamic integrity is related to structural abnormalities observed across the cortex and poor clinical outcomes [284, 285]. It has been reported that 40 h of TCT increased the left thalamic volume in subjects with early schizophrenia, and this increase significantly correlated with improvements in neurocognition [286]. In addition, schizophrenic patients showed impaired working memory, hypoactivation in left middle frontal gyri. After 80 h of CBT, they improved their working memory performance and showed increased activation in left middle frontal gyri. They also demonstrated a significant association between enhanced task performance and right middle frontal gyri signal, similar to healthy controls [287]. These data suggest a possible neuroprotective effect of CBT that might rescue the cognitive deficits in schizophreina.

Exercise can induce plasticity and promote learning and memory formation. As mentioned before, BDNF is involved in synaptic plasticity and probably mediates the effects of many psychiatric treatments. Actually, physical exercise increases *Bdnf* expression in rat hippocampus [288], and exercise-induced plasticity is also dependent on *Bdnf* signaling. During exercise, muscles release metabolite lactate, which can cross the blood-brain-barrier, activate Sirtuin1 deacetylase, which in turn increases the levels of the transcriptional coactivator PGC1a and the secreted molecule FNDC5 that mediate Bdnf expression, and finally upregulate Bdnf level and the downstream TrkB signaling in the hippocampus [289]. Thus, exercise can improve cognition via enhancing BDNF function and could be an effective conjunctive therapy for cognitive deficits in neurodegenerative disorders like Alzheimer's disease.

6. Conclusion

Pathological synaptic plasticity plays a crucial role in the development and progression of various neurological disorders. It can result from genetic mutations, environmental factors, and protein misfolding. For instance, in Alzheimer's disease, synaptic dysfunction and loss are driven by Aβ and tau proteins. In Parkinson's disease, changes in synaptic plasticity in the basal ganglia and dopamine dysregulation are key factors. Epilepsy involves hyperexcitability and neurotransmitter imbalances, while schizophrenia is marked by altered synaptic connectivity and NMDAR hypofunction. Autism spectrum disorders involve abnormal synaptic plasticity and genetic mutations affecting synaptic proteins.

Author details

CongYu Jin* and Kaj Karlstedt
Department of Physiology, Medicum, University of Helsinki, Finland

*Address all correspondence to: congyu.jin@helsinki.fi

References

[1] Hughes JR. Post-tetanic potentiation. Physiological Reviews. 1958;**38**(1):91-113. DOI: 10.1152/physrev.1958.38.1.91

[2] Malenka RC, Bear MF. LTP and LTD: An embarrassment of riches. Neuron. 2004;**44**(1):5-21. DOI: 10.1016/j.neuron.2004.09.012

[3] Kandel ER, Dudai Y, Mayford MR. The molecular and systems biology of memory. Cell. 2014;**157**(1):163-186. DOI: 10.1016/j.cell.2014.03.001

[4] Nabavi S, Fox R, Proulx CD, Lin JY, Tsien RY, Malinow R. Engineering a memory with LTD and LTP. Nature. 2014;**511**(7509):348-352. DOI: 10.1038/nature13294. Epub 2014 Jun 1

[5] Bliss TV, Lomo T. Long-lasting potentiation of synaptic transmission in the dentate area of the anaesthetized rabbit following stimulation of the perforant path. The Journal of Physiology. 1973;**232**(2):331-356. DOI: 10.1113/jphysiol.1973.sp010273

[6] Barrionuevo G, Schottler F, Lynch G. The effects of repetitive low frequency stimulation on control and "potentiated" synaptic responses in the hippocampus. Life Sciences. 1980;**27**(24):2385-2391. DOI: 10.1016/0024-3205(80)90509-3

[7] Dudek SM, Bear MF. Homosynaptic long-term depression in area CA1 of hippocampus and effects of N-methyl-D-aspartate receptor blockade. Proceedings of the National Academy of Sciences of the United States of America. 1992;**89**(10):4363-4367. DOI: 10.1073/pnas.89.10.4363

[8] Citri A, Malenka RC. Synaptic plasticity: Multiple forms, functions, and mechanisms. Neuropsychopharmacology. 2008;**33**(1):18-41. DOI: 10.1038/sj.npp.1301559

[9] Turrigiano GG, Nelson SB. Homeostatic plasticity in the developing nervous system. Nature Reviews. Neuroscience. 2004;**5**(2):97-107

[10] Shouval HZ. Models of synaptic plasticity. Scholarpedia. 2007;**2**:1605

[11] Bear MF, Abraham WC. Long-term depression in hippocampus. Annual Review of Neuroscience. 1996;**19**:437-462. DOI: 10.1146/annurev.ne.19.030196.002253

[12] Nicoll RA, Malenka RC. Contrasting properties of two forms of long-term potentiation in the hippocampus. Nature. 1995;**377**(6545):115-118. DOI: 10.1038/377115a0

[13] Linden DJ, Connor JA. Participation of postsynaptic PKC in cerebellar long-term depression in culture. Science. 1991;**254**(5038):1656-1659. DOI: 10.1126/science.1721243

[14] De Zeeuw CI, Hansel C, Bian F, Koekkoek SK, van Alphen AM, Linden DJ, et al. Expression of a protein kinase C inhibitor in Purkinje cells blocks cerebellar LTD and adaptation of the vestibulo-ocular reflex. Neuron. 1998;**20**(3):495-508. DOI: 10.1016/s0896-6273(00)80990-3

[15] Bellone C, Lüscher C. mGluRs induce a long-term depression in the ventral tegmental area that involves a switch of the subunit composition of AMPA receptors. The European Journal of Neuroscience. 2005;**21**(5):1280-1288. DOI: 10.1111/j.1460-9568.2005.03979.x

[16] Huang CC, Hsu KS. Sustained activation of metabotropic glutamate receptor 5 and protein tyrosine phosphatases mediate the expression of (S)-3,5-dihydroxyphenylglycine-induced long-term depression in the hippocampal CA1 region. Journal of Neurochemistry. 2006;**96**(1):179-194. DOI: 10.1111/j.1471-4159.2005.03527.x

[17] Hou L, Klann E. Activation of the phosphoinositide 3-kinase-Akt-mammalian target of rapamycin signaling pathway is required for metabotropic glutamate receptor-dependent long-term depression. The Journal of Neuroscience. 2004;**24**(28):6352-6361. DOI: 10.1523/JNEUROSCI.0995-04.2004

[18] Huber KM, Kayser MS, Bear MF. Role for rapid dendritic protein synthesis in hippocampal mGluR-dependent long-term depression. Science. 2000;**288**(5469):1254-1257. DOI: 10.1126/science.288.5469.1254

[19] Huber KM, Roder JC, Bear MF. Chemical induction of mGluR5- and protein synthesis–dependent long-term depression in hippocampal area CA1. Journal of Neurophysiology. 2001;**86**(1):321-325. DOI: 10.1152/jn.2001.86.1.321

[20] Snyder EM, Philpot BD, Huber KM, Dong X, Fallon JR, Bear MF. Internalization of ionotropic glutamate receptors in response to mGluR activation. Nature Neuroscience. 2001;**4**(11):1079-1085. DOI: 10.1038/nn746

[21] Ito M. Long-term depression. Annual Review of Neuroscience. 1989;**12**:85-102. DOI: 10.1146/annurev.ne.12.030189.000505

[22] Linden DJ, Connor JA. Long-term synaptic depression. Annual Review of Neuroscience. 1995;**18**:319-357. DOI: 10.1146/annurev.ne.18.030195.001535

[23] Huganir RL, Nicoll RA. AMPARs and synaptic plasticity: The last 25 years. Neuron. 2013;**80**(3):704-717. DOI: 10.1016/j.neuron.2013.10.025

[24] Gerdeman GL, Ronesi J, Lovinger DM. Postsynaptic endocannabinoid release is critical to long-term depression in the striatum. Nature Neuroscience. 2002;**5**(5):446-451. DOI: 10.1038/nn832

[25] Robbe D, Alonso G, Chaumont S, Bockaert J, Manzoni OJ. Role of p/q-Ca2+ channels in metabotropic glutamate receptor 2/3-dependent presynaptic long-term depression at nucleus accumbens synapses. The Journal of Neuroscience. 2002;**22**(11):4346-4356. DOI: 10.1523/JNEUROSCI.22-11-04346.2002

[26] Sjöström PJ, Turrigiano GG, Nelson SB. Neocortical LTD via coincident activation of presynaptic NMDA and cannabinoid receptors. Neuron. 2003;**39**(4):641-654. DOI: 10.1016/s0896-6273(03)00476-8

[27] Safo PK, Regehr WG. Endocannabinoids control the induction of cerebellar LTD. Neuron. 2005;**48**(4):647-659. DOI: 10.1016/j.neuron.2005.09.020

[28] Chevaleyre V, Takahashi KA, Castillo PE. Endocannabinoid-mediated synaptic plasticity in the CNS. Annual Review of Neuroscience. 2006;**29**:37-76. DOI: 10.1146/annurev.neuro.29.051605.112834

[29] Viveros MP, Marco EM, Llorente R, López-Gallardo M. Endocannabinoid system and synaptic plasticity: Implications for emotional responses. Neural Plasticity. 2007;**2007**:52908. DOI: 10.1155/2007/52908

[30] Mulkey RM, Malenka RC. Mechanisms underlying induction of homosynaptic long-term depression in area CA1 of the hippocampus. Neuron. 1992;**9**(5):967-975. DOI: 10.1016/0896-6273(92)90248-c

[31] Aiba A, Kano M, Chen C, Stanton ME, Fox GD, Herrup K, et al. Deficient cerebellar long-term depression and impaired motor learning in mGluR1 mutant mice. Cell. 1994;**79**(2):377-388

[32] Shigemoto R, Abe T, Nomura S, Nakanishi S, Hirano T. Antibodies inactivating mGluR1 metabotropic glutamate receptor block long-term depression in cultured Purkinje cells. Neuron. 1994;**12**(6):1245-1255. DOI: 10.1016/0896-6273(94)90441-3

[33] Yasuda H, Barth AL, Stellwagen D, Malenka RC. A developmental switch in the signaling cascades for LTP induction. Nature Neuroscience. 2003;**6**(1):15-16. DOI: 10.1038/nn985

[34] Malenka RC, Nicoll RA. Long-term potentiation–a decade of progress? Science. 1999;**285**(5435):1870-1874. DOI: 10.1126/science.285.5435.1870

[35] Bliss TV, Collingridge GL. A synaptic model of memory: Long-term potentiation in the hippocampus. Nature. 1993;**361**(6407):31-39. DOI: 10.1038/361031a0

[36] Malenka RC, Kauer JA, Zucker RS, Nicoll RA. Postsynaptic calcium is sufficient for potentiation of hippocampal synaptic transmission. Science. 1988;**242**(4875):81-84. DOI: 10.1126/science.2845577

[37] Yang SN, Tang YG, Zucker RS. Selective induction of LTP and LTD by postsynaptic [Ca2+]i elevation. Journal of Neurophysiology. 1999;**81**(2):781-787. DOI: 10.1152/jn.1999.81.2.781

[38] Derkach V, Barria A, Soderling TR. Ca^{2+}/calmodulin-kinase II enhances channel conductance of alpha-amino-3-hydroxy-5-methyl-4-isoxazolepropionate type glutamate receptors. Proceedings of the National Academy of Sciences of the United States of America. 1999;**96**:3269-3274

[39] Derkach VA, Oh MC, Guire ES, Soderling TR. Regulatory mechanisms of AMPA receptors in synaptic plasticity. Nature Reviews. Neuroscience. 2007;**8**(2):101-113. DOI: 10.1038/nrn2055

[40] Esteban JA, Shi SH, Wilson C, Nuriya M, Huganir RL, Malinow R. PKA phosphorylation of AMPA receptor subunits controls synaptic trafficking underlying plasticity. Nature Neuroscience. 2003;**6**(2):136-143. DOI: 10.1038/nn997

[41] Park AJ, Havekes R, Choi JH, Luczak V, Nie T, Huang T, et al. A presynaptic role for PKA in synaptic tagging and memory. Neurobiology of Learning and Memory. 2014;**114**:101-112. DOI: 10.1016/j.nlm.2014.05.005

[42] Abbott LF, Regehr WG. Synaptic computation. Nature. 2004;**431**(7010):796-803. DOI: 10.1038/nature03010

[43] Hennig MH. Theoretical models of synaptic short term plasticity. Frontiers in Computational Neuroscience. 2013;7:45. DOI: 10.3389/fncom.2013.00045

[44] Appelbaum LG, Shenasa MA, Stolz L, Daskalakis Z. Synaptic plasticity and mental health: Methods, challenges and opportunities. Neuropsychopharmacology. 2023;**48**(1):113-120. DOI: 10.1038/s41386-022-01370-w

[45] Skaper SD, Facci L, Zusso M, Giusti P. Synaptic plasticity, dementia

and Alzheimer disease. CNS & Neurological Disorders Drug Targets. 2017;**16**(3):220-233. DOI: 10.2174/1871527316666170113120853

[46] DeKosky ST, Scheff SW. Synapse loss in frontal cortex biopsies in Alzheimer's disease: Correlation with cognitive severity. Annals of Neurology. 1990;**27**(5):457-464. DOI: 10.1002/ana.410270502

[47] Terry RD, Masliah E, Salmon DP, Butters N, DeTeresa R, Hill R, et al. Physical basis of cognitive alterations in Alzheimer's disease: Synapse loss is the major correlate of cognitive impairment. Annals of Neurology. 1991;**30**(4):572-580. DOI: 10.1002/ana.410300410

[48] Selkoe DJ. Alzheimer's disease is a synaptic failure. Science. 2002;**298**(5594):789-791. DOI: 10.1126/science.1074069

[49] Honer WG. Pathology of presynaptic proteins in Alzheimer's disease: More than simple loss of terminals. Neurobiology of Aging. 2003;**24**(8):1047-1062. DOI: 10.1016/j.neurobiolaging.2003.04.005

[50] Palop JJ, Chin J, Mucke L. A network dysfunction perspective on neurodegenerative diseases. Nature. 2006;**443**(7113):768-773. DOI: 10.1038/nature05289

[51] Meftah S, Gan J. Alzheimer's disease as a synaptopathy: Evidence for dysfunction of synapses during disease progression. Frontiers in Synaptic Neuroscience. 2023;**15**:1129036. DOI: 10.3389/fnsyn.2023.1129036

[52] Shaw P, Lerch JP, Pruessner JC, Taylor KN, Rose AB, Greenstein D, et al. Cortical morphology in children and adolescents with different apolipoprotein E gene polymorphisms: An observational study. Lancet Neurology. 2007;**6**(6):494-500. DOI: 10.1016/S1474-4422(07)70106-0

[53] Domínguez-Álvaro M, Montero-Crespo M, Blazquez-Llorca L, DeFelipe J, Alonso-Nanclares L. 3D electron microscopy study of synaptic organization of the normal human transentorhinal cortex and its possible alterations in Alzheimer's disease. eNeuro. 2019;**6**(4):ENEURO.0140-19.2019. DOI: 10.1523/ENEURO.0140-19.2019

[54] Jacob CP, Koutsilieri E, Bartl J, Neuen-Jacob E, Arzberger T, Zander N, et al. Alterations in expression of glutamatergic transporters and receptors in sporadic Alzheimer's disease. Journal of Alzheimer's Disease. 2007;**11**(1):97-116. DOI: 10.3233/jad-2007-11113

[55] Gong Y, Lippa CF, Zhu J, Lin Q, Rosso AL. Disruption of glutamate receptors at shank-postsynaptic platform in Alzheimer's disease. Brain Research. 2009;**1292**:191-198. DOI: 10.1016/j.brainres.2009.07.056. Epub 2009 Jul 25

[56] Marcello E, Epis R, Saraceno C, Gardoni F, Borroni B, Cattabeni F, et al. SAP97-mediated local trafficking is altered in Alzheimer disease patients' hippocampus. Neurobiology of Aging. 2012;**33**(2):422.e1-422.10. DOI: 10.1016/j.neurobiolaging.2010.09.015

[57] Sze C, Bi H, Kleinschmidt-DeMasters BK, Filley CM, Martin LJ. N-methyl-D-aspartate receptor subunit proteins and their phosphorylation status are altered selectively in Alzheimer's disease. Journal of the Neurological Sciences. 2001;**182**(2):151-159. DOI: 10.1016/s0022-510x(00)00467-6

[58] Bi H, Sze CI. N-methyl-D-aspartate receptor subunit NR2A and NR2B

messenger RNA levels are altered in the hippocampus and entorhinal cortex in Alzheimer's disease. Journal of the Neurological Sciences. 2002;**200**(1-2):11-18. DOI: 10.1016/s0022-510x(02)00087-4

[59] Mishizen-Eberz AJ, Rissman RA, Carter TL, Ikonomovic MD, Wolfe BB, Armstrong DM. Biochemical and molecular studies of NMDA receptor subunits NR1/2A/2B in hippocampal subregions throughout progression of Alzheimer's disease pathology. Neurobiology of Disease. 2004;**15**(1):80-92. DOI: 10.1016/j.nbd.2003.09.016

[60] Romanelli MF, Morris JC, Ashkin K, Coben LA. Advanced Alzheimer's disease is a risk factor for late-onset seizures. Archives of Neurology. 1990;**47**(8):847-850. DOI: 10.1001/archneur.1990.00530080029006

[61] Irizarry MC, Jin S, He F, Emond JA, Raman R, Thomas RG, et al. Incidence of new-onset seizures in mild to moderate Alzheimer disease. Archives of Neurology. 2012;**69**(3):368-372. DOI: 10.1001/archneurol.2011.830

[62] Nicastro N, Assal F, Seeck M. From here to epilepsy: The risk of seizure in patients with Alzheimer's disease. Epileptic Disorders. 2016;**18**(1):1-12. DOI: 10.1684/epd.2016.0808

[63] Li S, Selkoe DJ. A mechanistic hypothesis for the impairment of synaptic plasticity by soluble Aβ oligomers from Alzheimer's brain. Journal of Neurochemistry. 2020;**154**(6):583-597. DOI: 10.1111/jnc.15007

[64] Schirinzi T, Canevelli M, Suppa A, Bologna M, Marsili L. The continuum between neurodegeneration, brain plasticity, and movement: A critical appraisal. Reviews in the Neurosciences. 2020;**31**(7):723-742. DOI: 10.1515/revneuro-2020-0011

[65] Kawabata S. Excessive/aberrant and maladaptive synaptic plasticity: A hypothesis for the pathogenesis of Alzheimer's disease. Frontiers in Aging Neuroscience. 2022;**14**:913693. DOI: 10.3389/fnagi.2022.913693

[66] Latif-Hernandez A, Sabanov V, Ahmed T, Craessaerts K, Saito T, Saido T, et al. The two faces of synaptic failure in App^{NL-G-F} knock-in mice. Alzheimer's Research & Therapy. 2020;**12**(1):100. DOI: 10.1186/s13195-020-00667-6

[67] Arroyo-García LE, Isla AG, Andrade-Talavera Y, Balleza-Tapia H, Loera-Valencia R, Alvarez-Jimenez L, et al. Impaired spike-gamma coupling of area CA3 fast-spiking interneurons as the earliest functional impairment in the App^{NL-G-F} mouse model of Alzheimer's disease. Molecular Psychiatry. 2021;**26**(10):5557-5567. DOI: 10.1038/s41380-021-01257-0

[68] Puzzo D, Privitera L, Leznik E, Fà M, Staniszewski A, Palmeri A, et al. Picomolar amyloid-beta positively modulates synaptic plasticity and memory in hippocampus. The Journal of Neuroscience. 2008;**28**(53):14537-14545. DOI: 10.1523/JNEUROSCI.2692-08.2008

[69] Mehak SF, Shivakumar AB, Kumari S, Muralidharan B, Gangadharan G. Theta and gamma oscillatory dynamics in mouse models of Alzheimer's disease: A path to prospective therapeutic intervention. Neuroscience and Biobehavioral Reviews. 2022;**136**:104628. DOI: 10.1016/j.neubiorev.2022.104628

[70] Regan P, Piers T, Yi JH, Kim DH, Huh S, Park SJ, et al. Tau phosphorylation at serine 396 residue is required for hippocampal LTD. The Journal of

Neuroscience. 2015;**35**(12):4804-4812. DOI: 10.1523/JNEUROSCI.2842-14.2015

[71] Bejanin A, Schonhaut DR, La Joie R, Kramer JH, Baker SL, Sosa N, et al. Tau pathology and neurodegeneration contribute to cognitive impairment in Alzheimer's disease. Brain. 2017;**140**(12):3286-3300. DOI: 10.1093/brain/awx243

[72] Xia C, Makaretz SJ, Caso C, McGinnis S, Gomperts SN, Sepulcre J, et al. Association of In Vivo [18F] AV-1451 tau PET imaging results with cortical atrophy and symptoms in typical and atypical Alzheimer disease. JAMA Neurology. 2017;**74**(4):427-436. DOI: 10.1001/jamaneurol.2016.5755

[73] Eckermann K, Mocanu MM, Khlistunova I, Biernat J, Nissen A, Hofmann A, et al. The beta-propensity of tau determines aggregation and synaptic loss in inducible mouse models of tauopathy. The Journal of Biological Chemistry. 2007;**282**(43):31755-31765. DOI: 10.1074/jbc.M705282200

[74] Sahara N, Murayama M, Higuchi M, Suhara T, Takashima A. Biochemical distribution of tau protein in Synaptosomal fraction of transgenic mice expressing human P301L tau. Frontiers in Neurology. 2014;**5**:26. DOI: 10.3389/fneur.2014.00026

[75] Xia D, Li C, Götz J. Pseudophosphorylation of tau at distinct epitopes or the presence of the P301L mutation targets the microtubule-associated protein tau to dendritic spines. Biochimica et Biophysica Acta. 2015;**1852**(5):913-924. DOI: 10.1016/j.bbadis.2014.12.017

[76] Yoshiyama Y, Higuchi M, Zhang B, Huang SM, Iwata N, Saido TC, et al. Synapse loss and microglial activation precede tangles in a P301S tauopathy mouse model. Neuron. 2007;**53**(3):337-351. DOI: 10.1016/j.neuron.2007.01.010. Erratum in: Neuron. 2007;54(2):343-4

[77] Hill E, Karikari TK, Moffat KG, Richardson MJE, Wall MJ. Introduction of tau oligomers into cortical neurons alters action potential dynamics and disrupts synaptic transmission and plasticity. eNeuro. 2019;**6**(5):ENEURO.0166-19.2019. DOI: 10.1523/ENEURO.0166-19.2019

[78] Fá M, Puzzo D, Piacentini R, Staniszewski A, Zhang H, Baltrons MA, et al. Extracellular tau oligomers produce an immediate impairment of LTP and memory. Scientific Reports. 2016;**6**:19393. DOI: 10.1038/srep19393

[79] Puzzo D, Piacentini R, Fá M, Gulisano W, Li Puma DD, Staniszewski A, et al. LTP and memory impairment caused by extracellular Aβ and tau oligomers is APP-dependent. eLife. 2017;**6**:e26991. DOI: 10.7554/eLife.26991

[80] Sydow A, Van der Jeugd A, Zheng F, Ahmed T, Balschun D, Petrova O, et al. Tau-induced defects in synaptic plasticity, learning, and memory are reversible in transgenic mice after switching off the toxic tau mutant. The Journal of Neuroscience. 2011;**31**(7):2511-2525. DOI: 10.1523/JNEUROSCI.5245-10.2011

[81] Booth CA, Witton J, Nowacki J, Tsaneva-Atanasova K, Jones MW, Randall AD, et al. Altered intrinsic pyramidal neuron properties and pathway-specific synaptic dysfunction underlie aberrant hippocampal network function in a mouse model of Tauopathy. The Journal of Neuroscience. 2016;**36**(2):350-363. DOI: 10.1523/JNEUROSCI.2151-15.2016

[82] Taylor HBC, Emptage NJ, Jeans AF. Long-term depression links amyloid-β to

the pathological hyperphosphorylation of tau. Cell Reports. 2021;**36**(9):109638. DOI: 10.1016/j.celrep.2021.109638

[83] Sourkes TL, Poirier LJ. Neurochemical bases of tremor and other disorders of movement. Canadian Medical Association Journal. 1966;**94**(2):53-60

[84] Pearce J, Pearce I. Current concepts of parkinsonism. Postgraduate Medical Journal. 1971;**47**(554):794-799. DOI: 10.1136/pgmj.47.554.794

[85] Albin RL, Young AB, Penney JB. The functional anatomy of basal ganglia disorders. Trends in Neurosciences. 1989;**12**(10):366-375. DOI: 10.1016/0166-2236(89)90074-x

[86] Kreitzer AC, Malenka RC. Striatal plasticity and basal ganglia circuit function. Neuron. 2008;**60**(4):543-554. DOI: 10.1016/j.neuron.2008.11.005

[87] Pedrosa V, Clopath C. The role of neuromodulators in cortical plasticity. A computational perspective. Frontiers in Synaptic Neuroscience. 2017;**8**:38. DOI: 10.3389/fnsyn.2016.00038

[88] Gerfen CR, Engber TM, Mahan LC, Susel Z, Chase TN, Monsma FJ Jr, et al. D1 and D2 dopamine receptor-regulated gene expression of striatonigral and striatopallidal neurons. Science. 1990;**250**(4986):1429-1432. DOI: 10.1126/science.2147780

[89] Surmeier DJ, Graves SM, Shen W. Dopaminergic modulation of striatal networks in health and Parkinson's disease. Current Opinion in Neurobiology. 2014;**29**:109-117. DOI: 10.1016/j.conb.2014.07.008

[90] Mallet N, Ballion B, Le Moine C, Gonon F. Cortical inputs and GABA interneurons imbalance projection neurons in the striatum of parkinsonian rats. The Journal of Neuroscience. 2006;**26**(14):3875-3884. DOI: 10.1523/JNEUROSCI.4439-05.2006

[91] Ryan MB, Bair-Marshall C, Nelson AB. Aberrant striatal activity in parkinsonism and levodopa-induced dyskinesia. Cell Reports. 2018;**23**(12):3438-3446.e5. DOI: 10.1016/j.celrep.2018.05.059

[92] Escande MV, Taravini IR, Zold CL, Belforte JE, Murer MG. Loss of homeostasis in the direct pathway in a mouse model of asymptomatic Parkinson's disease. The Journal of Neuroscience. 2016;**36**(21):5686-5698. DOI: 10.1523/JNEUROSCI.0492-15.2016

[93] Parker PR, Lalive AL, Kreitzer AC. Pathway-specific remodeling of thalamostriatal synapses in parkinsonian mice. Neuron. 2016;**89**(4):734-740. DOI: 10.1016/j.neuron.2015.12.038

[94] Suarez LM, Solis O, Sanz-Magro A, Alberquilla S, Moratalla R. Dopamine D1 receptors regulate spines in striatal direct-pathway and indirect-pathway neurons. Movement Disorders. 2020;**35**(10):1810-1821. DOI: 10.1002/mds.28174

[95] Schwarzschild MA, Agnati L, Fuxe K, Chen JF, Morelli M. Targeting adenosine A2A receptors in Parkinson's disease. Trends in Neurosciences. 2006;**29**(11):647-654. DOI: 10.1016/j.tins.2006.09.004

[96] Shen W, Flajolet M, Greengard P, Surmeier DJ. Dichotomous dopaminergic control of striatal synaptic plasticity. Science. 2008;**321**(5890):848-851. DOI: 10.1126/science.1160575

[97] Thiele SL, Chen B, Lo C, Gertler TS, Warre R, Surmeier JD, et al. Selective loss of bi-directional synaptic

plasticity in the direct and indirect striatal output pathways accompanies generation of parkinsonism and l-DOPA induced dyskinesia in mouse models. Neurobiology of Disease. 2014;**71**:334-344. DOI: 10.1016/j.nbd.2014.08.006

[98] Chu HY. Synaptic and cellular plasticity in Parkinson's disease. Acta Pharmacologica Sinica. 2020;**41**(4):447-452. DOI: 10.1038/s41401-020-0371-0

[99] Kreitzer AC, Malenka RC. Endocannabinoid-mediated rescue of striatal LTD and motor deficits in Parkinson's disease models. Nature. 2007;**445**(7128):643-647. DOI: 10.1038/nature05506

[100] Shahmoradian SH, Lewis AJ, Genoud C, Hench J, Moors TE, Navarro PP, et al. Lewy pathology in Parkinson's disease consists of crowded organelles and lipid membranes. Nature Neuroscience. 2019;**22**(7):1099-1109. DOI: 10.1038/s41593-019-0423-2

[101] Lashuel HA. Do Lewy bodies contain alpha-synuclein fibrils? And does it matter? A brief history and critical analysis of recent reports. Neurobiology of Disease. 2020;**141**:104876. DOI: 10.1016/j.nbd.2020.104876

[102] Simón-Sánchez J, Schulte C, Bras JM, Sharma M, Gibbs JR, Berg D, et al. Genome-wide association study reveals genetic risk underlying Parkinson's disease. Nature Genetics. 2009;**41**(12):1308-1312. DOI: 10.1038/ng.487

[103] Albarran E, Sun Y, Liu Y, Raju K, Dong A, Li Y, et al. Postsynaptic synucleins mediate endocannabinoid signaling. Nature Neuroscience. 2023;**26**(6):997-1007. DOI: 10.1038/s41593-023-01345-0

[104] Lewis DA, Sweet RA. Schizophrenia from a neural circuitry perspective: Advancing toward rational pharmacological therapies. The Journal of Clinical Investigation. 2009;**119**(4):706-716. DOI: 10.1172/JCI37335

[105] Garey LJ, Ong WY, Patel TS, Kanani M, Davis A, Mortimer AM, et al. Reduced dendritic spine density on cerebral cortical pyramidal neurons in schizophrenia. Journal of Neurology, Neurosurgery, and Psychiatry. 1998;**65**(4):446-453. DOI: 10.1136/jnnp.65.4.446

[106] Glantz LA, Lewis DA. Decreased dendritic spine density on prefrontal cortical pyramidal neurons in schizophrenia. Archives of General Psychiatry. 2000;**57**(1):65-73. DOI: 10.1001/archpsyc.57.1.65

[107] Kolluri N, Sun Z, Sampson AR, Lewis DA. Lamina-specific reductions in dendritic spine density in the prefrontal cortex of subjects with schizophrenia. The American Journal of Psychiatry. 2005;**162**(6):1200-1202. DOI: 10.1176/appi.ajp.162.6.1200

[108] Jones EG. Cortical development and thalamic pathology in schizophrenia. Schizophrenia Bulletin. 1997;**23**(3):483-501. DOI: 10.1093/schbul/23.3.483

[109] Moghaddam B. Targeting metabotropic glutamate receptors for treatment of the cognitive symptoms of schizophrenia. Psychopharmacology. 2004;**174**(1):39-44. DOI: 10.1007/s00213-004-1792-z

[110] Patil ST, Zhang L, Martenyi F, Lowe SL, Jackson KA, Andreev BV, et al. Activation of mGlu2/3 receptors as a new approach to treat schizophrenia: A randomized phase 2 clinical trial. Nature Medicine. 2007;**13**(9):1102-1107. DOI: 10.1038/nm1632. Epub 2007 Sep 2. Erratum in: Nat Med. 2007 Oct;13(10):1264

[111] Crabtree GW, Gogos JA. Synaptic plasticity, neural circuits, and the emerging role of altered short-term information processing in schizophrenia. Frontiers in Synaptic Neuroscience. 2014;**6**:28. DOI: 10.3389/fnsyn.2014.00028

[112] Javitt DC, Zukin SR. Recent advances in the phencyclidine model of schizophrenia. The American Journal of Psychiatry. 1991;**148**(10):1301-1308. DOI: 10.1176/ajp.148.10.1301

[113] Krystal JH, Karper LP, Seibyl JP, Freeman GK, Delaney R, Bremner JD, et al. Subanesthetic effects of the noncompetitive NMDA antagonist, ketamine, in humans. Psychotomimetic, perceptual, cognitive, and neuroendocrine responses. Archives of General Psychiatry. 1994;**51**(3):199-214. DOI: 10.1001/archpsyc.1994.03950030035004

[114] Coyle JT. Glutamate and schizophrenia: Beyond the dopamine hypothesis. Cellular and Molecular Neurobiology. 2006;**26**(4-6):365-384. DOI: 10.1007/s10571-006-9062-8

[115] Dalmau J, Lancaster E, Martinez-Hernandez E, Rosenfeld MR, Balice-Gordon R. Clinical experience and laboratory investigations in patients with anti-NMDAR encephalitis. Lancet Neurology. 2011;**10**(1):63-74. DOI: 10.1016/S1474-4422(10)70253-2

[116] Al-Diwani A, Handel A, Townsend L, Pollak T, Leite MI, Harrison PJ, et al. The psychopathology of NMDAR-antibody encephalitis in adults: A systematic review and phenotypic analysis of individual patient data. Lancet Psychiatry. 2019;**6**(3):235-246. DOI: 10.1016/S2215-0366(19)30001-X

[117] Weickert CS, Fung SJ, Catts VS, Schofield PR, Allen KM, Moore LT, et al. Molecular evidence of N-methyl-D-aspartate receptor hypofunction in schizophrenia. Molecular Psychiatry. 2013;**18**(11):1185-1192. DOI: 10.1038/mp.2012.137

[118] Catts VS, Lai YL, Weickert CS, Weickert TW, Catts SV. A quantitative review of the postmortem evidence for decreased cortical N-methyl-D-aspartate receptor expression levels in schizophrenia: How can we link molecular abnormalities to mismatch negativity deficits? Biological Psychology. 2016;**116**:57-67. DOI: 10.1016/j.biopsycho.2015.10.013

[119] Banerjee A, Wang HY, Borgmann-Winter KE, MacDonald ML, Kaprielian H, Stucky A, et al. Src kinase as a mediator of convergent molecular abnormalities leading to NMDAR hypoactivity in schizophrenia. Molecular Psychiatry. 2015;**20**(9):1091-1100. DOI: 10.1038/mp.2014.115

[120] Gerber DJ, Hall D, Miyakawa T, Demars S, Gogos JA, Karayiorgou M, et al. Evidence for association of schizophrenia with genetic variation in the 8p21.3 gene, PPP3CC, encoding the calcineurin gamma subunit. Proceedings of the National Academy of Sciences of the United States of America. 2003;**100**(15):8993-8998. DOI: 10.1073/pnas.1432927100

[121] Miyakawa T, Leiter LM, Gerber DJ, Gainetdinov RR, Sotnikova TD, Zeng H, et al. Conditional calcineurin knockout mice exhibit multiple abnormal behaviors related to schizophrenia. Proceedings of the National Academy of Sciences of the United States of America. 2003;**100**(15):8987-8992. DOI: 10.1073/pnas.1432926100

[122] Du J, Gray NA, Falke C, Yuan P, Szabo S, Manji HK. Structurally dissimilar antimanic agents modulate

synaptic plasticity by regulating AMPA glutamate receptor subunit GluR1 synaptic expression. Annals of the New York Academy of Sciences. 2003;**1003**:378-380. DOI: 10.1196/annals.1300.031

[123] Du J, Gray NA, Falke CA, Chen W, Yuan P, Szabo ST, et al. Modulation of synaptic plasticity by antimanic agents: The role of AMPA glutamate receptor subunit 1 synaptic expression. The Journal of Neuroscience. 2004;**24**(29):6578-6589. DOI: 10.1523/JNEUROSCI.1258-04.2004

[124] Du J, Suzuki K, Wei Y, Wang Y, Blumenthal R, Chen Z, et al. The anticonvulsants lamotrigine, riluzole, and valproate differentially regulate AMPA receptor membrane localization: Relationship to clinical effects in mood disorders. Neuropsychopharmacology. 2007;**32**(4):793-802. DOI: 10.1038/sj.npp.1301178

[125] Compte A, Brunel N, Goldman-Rakic PS, Wang XJ. Synaptic mechanisms and network dynamics underlying spatial working memory in a cortical network model. Cerebral Cortex. 2000;**10**(9):910-923. DOI: 10.1093/cercor/10.9.910

[126] Mongillo G, Barak O, Tsodyks M. Synaptic theory of working memory. Science. 2008;**319**(5869):1543-1546. DOI: 10.1126/science.1150769

[127] Frankle WG, Lerma J, Laruelle M. The synaptic hypothesis of schizophrenia. Neuron. 2003;**39**(2):205-216. DOI: 10.1016/s0896-6273(03)00423-9

[128] Xu B, Ionita-Laza I, Roos JL, Boone B, Woodrick S, Sun Y, et al. De novo gene mutations highlight patterns of genetic and neural complexity in schizophrenia. Nature Genetics. 2012;**44**(12):1365-1369. DOI: 10.1038/ng.2446

[129] Paterlini M, Zakharenko SS, Lai WS, Qin J, Zhang H, Mukai J, et al. Transcriptional and behavioral interaction between 22q11.2 orthologs modulates schizophrenia-related phenotypes in mice. Nature Neuroscience. 2005;**8**(11):1586-1594. DOI: 10.1038/nn1562

[130] Millar JK, Wilson-Annan JC, Anderson S, Christie S, Taylor MS, Semple CA, et al. Disruption of two novel genes by a translocation co-segregating with schizophrenia. Human Molecular Genetics. 2000;**9**(9):1415-1423. DOI: 10.1093/hmg/9.9.1415

[131] Blackwood DH, Fordyce A, Walker MT, St. Clair DM, Porteous DJ, Muir WJ. Schizophrenia and affective disorders–cosegregation with a translocation at chromosome 1q42 that directly disrupts brain-expressed genes: Clinical and P300 findings in a family. American Journal of Human Genetics. 2001;**69**(2):428-433. DOI: 10.1086/321969

[132] Bradshaw NJ, Trossbach SV, Köber S, Walter S, Prikulis I, Weggen S, et al. Disrupted in schizophrenia 1 regulates the processing of reelin in the perinatal cortex. Schizophrenia Research. 2020;**215**:506-513. DOI: 10.1016/j.schres.2017.04.012

[133] Lakatosova S, Ostatnikova D. Reelin and its complex involvement in brain development and function. The International Journal of Biochemistry & Cell Biology. 2012;**44**(9):1501-1504. DOI: 10.1016/j.biocel.2012.06.002

[134] Pantazopoulos H, Berretta S. In sickness and in health: Perineuronal nets and synaptic plasticity in psychiatric disorders. Neural

Plasticity. 2016;**2016**:9847696. DOI: 10.1155/2016/9847696

[135] Dityatev A, Seidenbecher CI, Schachner M. Compartmentalization from the outside: The extracellular matrix and functional microdomains in the brain. Trends in Neurosciences. 2010;**33**(11):503-512. DOI: 10.1016/j.tins.2010.08.003

[136] Schell MJ, Molliver ME, Snyder SH. D-serine, an endogenous synaptic modulator: Localization to astrocytes and glutamate-stimulated release. Proceedings of the National Academy of Sciences of the United States of America. 1995;**92**(9):3948-3952. DOI: 10.1073/pnas.92.9.3948

[137] Lepeta K, Lourenco MV, Schweitzer BC, Martino Adami PV, Banerjee P, Catuara-Solarz S, et al. Synaptopathies: Synaptic dysfunction in neurological disorders - A review from students to students. Journal of Neurochemistry. 2016;**138**(6):785-805. DOI: 10.1111/jnc.13713

[138] Qiu S, Zhao LF, Korwek KM, Weeber EJ. Differential reelin-induced enhancement of NMDA and AMPA receptor activity in the adult hippocampus. The Journal of Neuroscience. 2006;**26**(50):12943-12955. DOI: 10.1523/JNEUROSCI.2561-06.2006

[139] Förster E, Bock HH, Herz J, Chai X, Frotscher M, Zhao S. Emerging topics in Reelin function. The European Journal of Neuroscience. 2010;**31**(9):1511-1518. DOI: 10.1111/j.1460-9568.2010.07222.x

[140] Dityatev A, Schachner M, Sonderegger P. The dual role of the extracellular matrix in synaptic plasticity and homeostasis. Nature Reviews. Neuroscience. 2010;**11**(11):735-746. DOI: 10.1038/nrn2898

[141] Pozo K, Goda Y. Unraveling mechanisms of homeostatic synaptic plasticity. Neuron. 2010;**66**(3):337-351. DOI: 10.1016/j.neuron.2010.04.028

[142] Frischknecht R, Heine M, Perrais D, Seidenbecher CI, Choquet D, Gundelfinger ED. Brain extracellular matrix affects AMPA receptor lateral mobility and short-term synaptic plasticity. Nature Neuroscience. 2009;**12**(7):897-904. DOI: 10.1038/nn.2338

[143] Bukalo O, Schachner M, Dityatev A. Modification of extracellular matrix by enzymatic removal of chondroitin sulfate and by lack of tenascin-R differentially affects several forms of synaptic plasticity in the hippocampus. Neuroscience. 2001;**104**(2):359-369. DOI: 10.1016/s0306-4522(01)00082-3

[144] Earls LR, Zakharenko SS. A synaptic function approach to investigating complex psychiatric diseases. The Neuroscientist. 2014;**20**(3):257-271. DOI: 10.1177/1073858413498307

[145] Bitanihirwe BK, Mauney SA, Woo TU. Weaving a net of neurobiological mechanisms in schizophrenia and Unraveling the underlying pathophysiology. Biological Psychiatry. 2016;**80**(8):589-598. DOI: 10.1016/j.biopsych.2016.03.1047

[146] Levy AD, Omar MH, Koleske AJ. Extracellular matrix control of dendritic spine and synapse structure and plasticity in adulthood. Frontiers in Neuroanatomy. 2014;**8**:116. DOI: 10.3389/fnana.2014.00116

[147] Mundy P. Annotation: The neural basis of social impairments in autism: The role of the dorsal medial-frontal cortex and anterior cingulate system. Journal of Child Psychology and

Psychiatry. 2003;**44**(6):793-809. DOI: 10.1111/1469-7610.00165

[148] Belmonte MK, Allen G, Beckel-Mitchener A, Boulanger LM, Carper RA, Webb SJ. Autism and abnormal development of brain connectivity. The Journal of Neuroscience. 2004;**24**(42):9228-9231. DOI: 10.1523/JNEUROSCI.3340-04.2004

[149] Rinaldi T, Kulangara K, Antoniello K, Markram H. Elevated NMDA receptor levels and enhanced postsynaptic long-term potentiation induced by prenatal exposure to valproic acid. Proceedings of the National Academy of Sciences of the United States of America. 2007;**104**(33):13501-13506. DOI: 10.1073/pnas.0704391104

[150] Rinaldi T, Perrodin C, Markram H. Hyper-connectivity and hyper-plasticity in the medial prefrontal cortex in the valproic acid animal model of autism. Frontiers in Neural Circuits. 2008;**2**:4. DOI: 10.3389/neuro.04.004.2008

[151] Rinaldi T, Silberberg G, Markram H. Hyperconnectivity of local neocortical microcircuitry induced by prenatal exposure to valproic acid. Cerebral Cortex. 2008;**18**(4):763-770. DOI: 10.1093/cercor/bhm117

[152] Markram K, Markram H. The intense world theory - A unifying theory of the neurobiology of autism. Frontiers in Human Neuroscience. 2010;**4**:224. DOI: 10.3389/fnhum.2010.00224

[153] Ecker C, Murphy D. Neuroimaging in autism–from basic science to translational research. Nature Reviews. Neurology. 2014;**10**(2):82-91. DOI: 10.1038/nrneurol.2013.276

[154] Mansour Y, Ahmed SN, Kulesza R. Abnormal morphology and subcortical projections to the medial geniculate in an animal model of autism. Experimental Brain Research. 2021;**239**(2):381-400. DOI: 10.1007/s00221-020-05982-w

[155] Park BY, Hong SJ, Valk SL, Paquola C, Benkarim O, Bethlehem RAI, et al. Differences in subcortico-cortical interactions identified from connectome and microcircuit models in autism. Nature Communications. 2021;**12**(1):2225. DOI: 10.1038/s41467-021-21732-0

[156] Arguello PA, Gogos JA. Genetic and cognitive windows into circuit mechanisms of psychiatric disease. Trends in Neurosciences. 2012;**35**(1):3-13. DOI: 10.1016/j.tins.2011.11.007

[157] Fu YH, Kuhl DP, Pizzuti A, Pieretti M, Sutcliffe JS, Richards S, et al. Variation of the CGG repeat at the fragile X site results in genetic instability: Resolution of the Sherman paradox. Cell. 1991;**67**(6):1047-1058. DOI: 10.1016/0092-8674(91)90283-5

[158] Verkerk AJ, Pieretti M, Sutcliffe JS, Fu YH, Kuhl DP, Pizzuti A, et al. Identification of a gene (FMR-1) containing a CGG repeat coincident with a breakpoint cluster region exhibiting length variation in fragile X syndrome. Cell. 1991;**65**(5):905-914. DOI: 10.1016/0092-8674(91)90397-h

[159] Amir RE, Van den Veyver IB, Wan M, Tran CQ, Francke U, Zoghbi HY. Rett syndrome is caused by mutations in X-linked MECP2, encoding methyl-CpG-binding protein 2. Nature Genetics. 1999;**23**(2):185-188. DOI: 10.1038/13810

[160] Bonaglia MC, Giorda R, Borgatti R, Felisari G, Gagliardi C, Selicorni A, et al. Disruption of the ProSAP2 gene in a t(12;22)(q24.1;q13.3) is associated with the 22q13.3 deletion syndrome. American Journal of Human

Genetics. 2001;**69**(2):261-268. DOI: 10.1086/321293. Epub 2001 Jun 18

[161] O'Donnell WT, Warren ST. A decade of molecular studies of fragile X syndrome. Annual Review of Neuroscience. 2002;**25**:315-338. DOI: 10.1146/annurev.neuro.25.112701.142909

[162] Qin M, Kang J, Burlin TV, Jiang C, Smith CB. Postadolescent changes in regional cerebral protein synthesis: An in vivo study in the FMR1 null mouse. The Journal of Neuroscience. 2005;**25**(20):5087-5095. DOI: 10.1523/JNEUROSCI.0093-05.2005

[163] Osterweil EK, Krueger DD, Reinhold K, Bear MF. Hypersensitivity to mGluR5 and ERK1/2 leads to excessive protein synthesis in the hippocampus of a mouse model of fragile X syndrome. The Journal of Neuroscience. 2010;**30**(46):15616-15627. DOI: 10.1523/JNEUROSCI.3888-10.2010

[164] Huber KM, Gallagher SM, Warren ST, Bear MF. Altered synaptic plasticity in a mouse model of fragile X mental retardation. Proceedings of the National Academy of Sciences of the United States of America. 2002;**99**(11):7746-7750. DOI: 10.1073/pnas.122205699

[165] Greenough WT, Klintsova AY, Irwin SA, Galvez R, Bates KE, Weiler IJ. Synaptic regulation of protein synthesis and the fragile X protein. Proceedings of the National Academy of Sciences of the United States of America. 2001;**98**(13):7101-7106. DOI: 10.1073/pnas.141145998

[166] Bear MF, Huber KM, Warren ST. The mGluR theory of fragile X mental retardation. Trends in Neurosciences. 2004;**27**(7):370-377. DOI: 10.1016/j.tins.2004.04.009

[167] Fyke W, Velinov M. *FMR1* and autism, an intriguing connection revisited. Genes (Basel). 2021;**12**(8):1218. DOI: 10.3390/genes12081218

[168] Zoghbi HY, Bear MF. Synaptic dysfunction in neurodevelopmental disorders associated with autism and intellectual disabilities. Cold Spring Harbor Perspectives in Biology. 2012;**4**(3):a009886. DOI: 10.1101/cshperspect.a009886

[169] Neul JL, Fang P, Barrish J, Lane J, Caeg EB, Smith EO, et al. Specific mutations in methyl-CpG-binding protein 2 confer different severity in Rett syndrome. Neurology. 2008;**70**(16):1313-1321. DOI: 10.1212/01.wnl.0000291011.54508.aa

[170] Lewis JD, Meehan RR, Henzel WJ, Maurer-Fogy I, Jeppesen P, Klein F, et al. Purification, sequence, and cellular localization of a novel chromosomal protein that binds to methylated DNA. Cell. 1992;**69**(6):905-914. DOI: 10.1016/0092-8674(92)90610-o

[171] Jones PL, Veenstra GJ, Wade PA, Vermaak D, Kass SU, Landsberger N, et al. Methylated DNA and MeCP2 recruit histone deacetylase to repress transcription. Nature Genetics. 1998;**19**(2):187-191. DOI: 10.1038/561

[172] Nan X, Ng HH, Johnson CA, Laherty CD, Turner BM, Eisenman RN, et al. Transcriptional repression by the methyl-CpG-binding protein MeCP2 involves a histone deacetylase complex. Nature. 1998;**393**(6683):386-389. DOI: 10.1038/30764

[173] Chen WG, Chang Q, Lin Y, Meissner A, West AE, Griffith EC, et al. Derepression of BDNF transcription involves calcium-dependent phosphorylation of MeCP2. Science.

2003;**302**(5646):885-889. DOI: 10.1126/science.1086446

[174] Martinowich K, Hattori D, Wu H, Fouse S, He F, Hu Y, et al. DNA methylation-related chromatin remodeling in activity-dependent BDNF gene regulation. Science. 2003;**302**(5646):890-893. DOI: 10.1126/science.1090842

[175] Yasui DH, Peddada S, Bieda MC, Vallero RO, Hogart A, Nagarajan RP, et al. Integrated epigenomic analyses of neuronal MeCP2 reveal a role for long-range interaction with active genes. Proceedings of the National Academy of Sciences of the United States of America. 2007;**104**(49):19416-19421. DOI: 10.1073/pnas.0707442104

[176] Chahrour M, Jung SY, Shaw C, Zhou X, Wong ST, Qin J, et al. MeCP2, a key contributor to neurological disease, activates and represses transcription. Science. 2008;**320**(5880):1224-1229. DOI: 10.1126/science.1153252

[177] Shahbazian MD, Antalffy B, Armstrong DL, Zoghbi HY. Insight into Rett syndrome: MeCP2 levels display tissue- and cell-specific differences and correlate with neuronal maturation. Human Molecular Genetics. 2002;**11**(2):115-124. DOI: 10.1093/hmg/11.2.115

[178] Maezawa I, Swanberg S, Harvey D, LaSalle JM, Jin LW. Rett syndrome astrocytes are abnormal and spread MeCP2 deficiency through gap junctions. The Journal of Neuroscience. 2009;**29**(16):5051-5061. DOI: 10.1523/JNEUROSCI.0324-09.2009

[179] Maezawa I, Jin LW. Rett syndrome microglia damage dendrites and synapses by the elevated release of glutamate. The Journal of Neuroscience. 2010;**30**(15):5346-5356. DOI: 10.1523/JNEUROSCI.5966-09.2010

[180] Kifayathullah LA, Arunachalam JP, Bodda C, Agbemenyah HY, Laccone FA, Mannan AU. MeCP2 mutant protein is expressed in astrocytes as well as in neurons and localizes in the nucleus. Cytogenetic and Genome Research. 2010;**129**(4):290-297. DOI: 10.1159/000315906

[181] Asaka Y, Jugloff DG, Zhang L, Eubanks JH, Fitzsimonds RM. Hippocampal synaptic plasticity is impaired in the Mecp2-null mouse model of Rett syndrome. Neurobiology of Disease. 2006;**21**(1):217-227. DOI: 10.1016/j.nbd.2005.07.005

[182] Moretti P, Levenson JM, Battaglia F, Atkinson R, Teague R, Antalffy B, et al. Learning and memory and synaptic plasticity are impaired in a mouse model of Rett syndrome. The Journal of Neuroscience. 2006;**26**(1):319-327. DOI: 10.1523/JNEUROSCI.2623-05.2006

[183] Collins AL, Levenson JM, Vilaythong AP, Richman R, Armstrong DL, Noebels JL, et al. Mild overexpression of MeCP2 causes a progressive neurological disorder in mice. Human Molecular Genetics. 2004;**13**(21):2679-2689. DOI: 10.1093/hmg/ddh282

[184] Ballas N, Lioy DT, Grunseich C, Mandel G. Non-cell autonomous influence of MeCP2-deficient glia on neuronal dendritic morphology. Nature Neuroscience. 2009;**12**(3):311-317. DOI: 10.1038/nn.2275

[185] Anderlid BM, Schoumans J, Annerén G, Tapia-Paez I, Dumanski J, Blennow E, et al. FISH-mapping of a 100-kb terminal 22q13 deletion. Human Genetics. 2002;**110**(5):439-443. DOI: 10.1007/s00439-002-0713-7

[186] Wilson HL, Wong AC, Shaw SR, Tse WY, Stapleton GA, Phelan MC,

et al. Molecular characterisation of the 22q13 deletion syndrome supports the role of haploinsufficiency of SHANK3/PROSAP2 in the major neurological symptoms. Journal of Medical Genetics. 2003;**40**(8):575-584. DOI: 10.1136/jmg.40.8.575

[187] Dhar SU, del Gaudio D, German JR, Peters SU, Ou Z, Bader PI, et al. 22q13.3 deletion syndrome: Clinical and molecular analysis using array CGH. American Journal of Medical Genetics. Part A. 2010;**152A**(3):573-581. DOI: 10.1002/ajmg.a.33253

[188] Durand CM, Betancur C, Boeckers TM, Bockmann J, Chaste P, Fauchereau F, et al. Mutations in the gene encoding the synaptic scaffolding protein SHANK3 are associated with autism spectrum disorders. Nature Genetics. 2007;**39**(1):25-27. DOI: 10.1038/ng1933

[189] Okamoto N, Kubota T, Nakamura Y, Murakami R, Nishikubo T, Tanaka I, et al. 22q13 microduplication in two patients with common clinical manifestations: A recognizable syndrome? American Journal of Medical Genetics. Part A. 2007;**143A**(23):2804-2809. DOI: 10.1002/ajmg.a.31771

[190] Roussignol G, Ango F, Romorini S, Tu JC, Sala C, Worley PF, et al. Shank expression is sufficient to induce functional dendritic spine synapses in aspiny neurons. The Journal of Neuroscience. 2005;**25**(14):3560-3570. DOI: 10.1523/JNEUROSCI.4354-04.2005

[191] Bozdagi O, Sakurai T, Papapetrou D, Wang X, Dickstein DL, Takahashi N, et al. Haploinsufficiency of the autism-associated Shank3 gene leads to deficits in synaptic function, social interaction, and social communication. Molecular Autism. 2010;**1**(1):15. DOI: 10.1186/2040-2392-1-15

[192] Arons MH, Thynne CJ, Grabrucker AM, Li D, Schoen M, Cheyne JE, et al. Autism-associated mutations in ProSAP2/Shank3 impair synaptic transmission and neurexin-neuroligin-mediated transsynaptic signaling. The Journal of Neuroscience. 2012;**32**(43):14966-14978. DOI: 10.1523/JNEUROSCI.2215-12.2012

[193] Autism Genome Project Consortium, Szatmari P, Paterson AD, Zwaigenbaum L, Roberts W, Brian J, et al. Mapping autism risk loci using genetic linkage and chromosomal rearrangements. Nature Genetics. 2007;**39**(3):319-328. DOI: 10.1038/ng1985

[194] Kim HG, Kishikawa S, Higgins AW, Seong IS, Donovan DJ, Shen Y, et al. Disruption of neurexin 1 associated with autism spectrum disorder. American Journal of Human Genetics. 2008;**82**(1):199-207. DOI: 10.1016/j.ajhg.2007.09.011

[195] Gauthier J, Siddiqui TJ, Huashan P, Yokomaku D, Hamdan FF, Champagne N, et al. Truncating mutations in NRXN2 and NRXN1 in autism spectrum disorders and schizophrenia. Human Genetics. 2011;**130**(4):563-573. DOI: 10.1007/s00439-011-0975-z

[196] Konopka G, Wexler E, Rosen E, Mukamel Z, Osborn GE, Chen L, et al. Modeling the functional genomics of autism using human neurons. Molecular Psychiatry. 2012;**17**(2):202-214. DOI: 10.1038/mp.2011.60

[197] Jamain S, Quach H, Betancur C, Råstam M, Colineaux C, Gillberg IC, et al. Mutations of the X-linked genes encoding neuroligins NLGN3 and NLGN4 are associated with autism. Nature Genetics. 2003;**34**(1):27-29. DOI: 10.1038/ng1136

[198] Südhof TC. Neuroligins and neurexins link synaptic function

to cognitive disease. Nature. 2008;**455**(7215):903-911. DOI: 10.1038/nature07456

[199] Tabuchi K, Blundell J, Etherton MR, Hammer RE, Liu X, Powell CM, et al. A neuroligin-3 mutation implicated in autism increases inhibitory synaptic transmission in mice. Science. 2007;**318**(5847):71-76. DOI: 10.1126/science.1146221

[200] Radyushkin K, Hammerschmidt K, Boretius S, Varoqueaux F, El-Kordi A, Ronnenberg A, et al. Neuroligin-3-deficient mice: Model of a monogenic heritable form of autism with an olfactory deficit. Genes, Brain, and Behavior. 2009;**8**(4):416-425. DOI: 10.1111/j.1601-183X.2009.00487.x

[201] Jamain S, Radyushkin K, Hammerschmidt K, Granon S, Boretius S, Varoqueaux F, et al. Reduced social interaction and ultrasonic communication in a mouse model of monogenic heritable autism. Proceedings of the National Academy of Sciences of the United States of America. 2008;**105**(5):1710-1715. DOI: 10.1073/pnas.0711555105

[202] Cavazos JE, Cross DJ. The role of synaptic reorganization in mesial temporal lobe epilepsy. Epilepsy & Behavior. 2006;**8**(3):483-493. DOI: 10.1016/j.yebeh.2006.01.011

[203] Engel J Jr. Update on surgical treatment of the epilepsies. Clinical and Experimental Neurology. 1992;**29**:32-48

[204] Babb TL, Lieb JP, Brown WJ, Pretorius J, Crandall PH. Distribution of pyramidal cell density and hyperexcitability in the epileptic human hippocampal formation. Epilepsia. 1984;**25**(6):721-728. DOI: 10.1111/j.1528-1157.1984.tb03483.x

[205] Wuarin JP, Dudek FE. Excitatory synaptic input to granule cells increases with time after kainate treatment. Journal of Neurophysiology. 2001;**85**(3):1067-1077. DOI: 10.1152/jn.2001.85.3.1067

[206] Okazaki MM, Molnár P, Nadler JV. Recurrent mossy fiber pathway in rat dentate gyrus: Synaptic currents evoked in presence and absence of seizure-induced growth. Journal of Neurophysiology. 1999;**81**(4):1645-1660. DOI: 10.1152/jn.1999.81.4.1645

[207] Scharfman HE, Sollas AL, Berger RE, Goodman JH. Electrophysiological evidence of monosynaptic excitatory transmission between granule cells after seizure-induced mossy fiber sprouting. Journal of Neurophysiology. 2003;**90**(4):2536-2547. DOI: 10.1152/jn.00251.2003

[208] Santhakumar V, Aradi I, Soltesz I. Role of mossy fiber sprouting and mossy cell loss in hyperexcitability: A network model of the dentate gyrus incorporating cell types and axonal topography. Journal of Neurophysiology. 2005;**93**(1):437-453. DOI: 10.1152/jn.00777.2004

[209] Kullmann DM, Asztely F, Walker MC. The role of mammalian ionotropic receptors in synaptic plasticity: LTP, LTD and epilepsy. Cellular and Molecular Life Sciences. 2000;**57**(11):1551-1561. DOI: 10.1007/pl00000640

[210] Mody I, Heinemann U. NMDA receptors of dentate gyrus granule cells participate in synaptic transmission following kindling. Nature. 1987;**326**(6114):701-704. DOI: 10.1038/326701a0

[211] Pratt GD, Kokaia M, Bengzon J, Kokaia Z, Fritschy JM, Möhler H, et al. Differential regulation of N-methyl-

D-aspartate receptor subunit messenger RNAs in kindling-induced epileptogenesis. Neuroscience. 1993;**57**(2):307-318. DOI: 10.1016/0306-4522(93)90064-m

[212] Pollard H, Héron A, Moreau J, Ben-Ari Y, Khrestchatisky M. Alterations of the GluR-B AMPA receptor subunit flip/flop expression in kainate-induced epilepsy and ischemia. Neuroscience. 1993;**57**(3):545-554. DOI: 10.1016/0306-4522(93)90004-y

[213] Friedman LK, Pellegrini-Giampietro DE, Sperber EF, Bennett MV, Moshé SL, Zukin RS. Kainate-induced status epilepticus alters glutamate and GABAA receptor gene expression in adult rat hippocampus: An in situ hybridization study. The Journal of Neuroscience. 1994;**14**(5 Pt. 1):2697-2707. DOI: 10.1523/JNEUROSCI.14-05-02697.1994

[214] Kamphuis W, De Rijk TC, Talamini LM, Lopes da Silva FH. Rat hippocampal kindling induces changes in the glutamate receptor mRNA expression patterns in dentate granule neurons. The European Journal of Neuroscience. 1994;**6**(7):1119-1127. DOI: 10.1111/j.1460-9568.1994.tb00609.x

[215] Kamphuis W, Hendriksen H, Diegenbach PC, Lopes da Silva FH. N-methyl-D-aspartate and kainate receptor gene expression in hippocampal pyramidal and granular neurons in the kindling model of epileptogenesis. Neuroscience. 1995;**67**(3):551-559. DOI: 10.1016/0306-4522(95)00070-y

[216] de Lanerolle NC, Eid T, von Campe G, Kovacs I, Spencer DD, Brines M. Glutamate receptor subunits GluR1 and GluR2/3 distribution shows reorganization in the human epileptogenic hippocampus. The European Journal of Neuroscience. 1998;**10**(5):1687-1703. DOI: 10.1046/j.1460-9568.1998.00171.x

[217] Köhr G, De Koninck Y, Mody I. Properties of NMDA receptor channels in neurons acutely isolated from epileptic (kindled) rats. The Journal of Neuroscience. 1993;**13**(8):3612-3627. DOI: 10.1523/JNEUROSCI.13-08-03612.1993

[218] Lieberman DN, Mody I. Regulation of NMDA channel function by endogenous Ca(2+)-dependent phosphatase. Nature. 1994;**369**(6477):235-239. DOI: 10.1038/369235a0

[219] Lieberman DN, Mody I. Properties of single NMDA receptor channels in human dentate gyrus granule cells. The Journal of Physiology. 1999;**518**(Pt. 1):55-70. DOI: 10.1111/j.1469-7793.1999.0055r.x

[220] Goodkin HP, Yeh JL, Kapur J. Status epilepticus increases the intracellular accumulation of GABAA receptors. The Journal of Neuroscience. 2005;**25**(23):5511-5520. DOI: 10.1523/JNEUROSCI.0900-05.2005

[221] Kapur J, Macdonald RL. Rapid seizure-induced reduction of benzodiazepine and Zn2+ sensitivity of hippocampal dentate granule cell GABAA receptors. The Journal of Neuroscience. 1997;**17**(19):7532-7540. DOI: 10.1523/JNEUROSCI.17-19-07532.1997

[222] Naylor DE, Liu H, Wasterlain CG. Trafficking of GABA(a) receptors, loss of inhibition, and a mechanism for pharmacoresistance in status epilepticus. The Journal of Neuroscience. 2005;**25**(34):7724-7733. DOI: 10.1523/JNEUROSCI.4944-04.2005

[223] Wasterlain CG, Liu H, Naylor DE, Thompson KW, Suchomelova L, Niquet J,

et al. Molecular basis of self-sustaining seizures and pharmacoresistance during status epilepticus: The receptor trafficking hypothesis revisited. Epilepsia. 2009;**50**(Suppl. 12):16-18. DOI: 10.1111/j.1528-1167.2009.02375.x

[224] Hwa GG, Avoli M. The involvement of excitatory amino acids in neocortical epileptogenesis: NMDA and non-NMDA receptors. Experimental Brain Research. 1991;**86**(2):248-256. DOI: 10.1007/BF00228949

[225] Traub RD, Miles R, Jefferys JG. Synaptic and intrinsic conductances shape picrotoxin-induced synchronized after-discharges in the Guinea-pig hippocampal slice. The Journal of Physiology. 1993;**461**:525-547. DOI: 10.1113/jphysiol.1993.sp019527

[226] Rogawski MA. AMPA receptors as a molecular target in epilepsy therapy. Acta Neurologica Scandinavica. Supplementum. 2013;**197**:9-18. DOI: 10.1111/ane.12099

[227] Rankin-Gee EK, McRae PA, Baranov E, Rogers S, Wandrey L, Porter BE. Perineuronal net degradation in epilepsy. Epilepsia. 2015;**56**(7):1124-1133. DOI: 10.1111/epi.13026

[228] Pollock E, Everest M, Brown A, Poulter MO. Metalloproteinase inhibition prevents inhibitory synapse reorganization and seizure genesis. Neurobiology of Disease. 2014;**70**:21-31. DOI: 10.1016/j.nbd.2014.06.003

[229] McRae PA, Porter BE. The perineuronal net component of the extracellular matrix in plasticity and epilepsy. Neurochemistry International. 2012;**61**(7):963-972. DOI: 10.1016/j.neuint.2012.08.007

[230] Seki T, Rutishauser U. Removal of polysialic acid-neural cell adhesion molecule induces aberrant mossy fiber innervation and ectopic synaptogenesis in the hippocampus. The Journal of Neuroscience. 1998;**18**(10):3757-3766. DOI: 10.1523/JNEUROSCI.18-10-03757.1998

[231] Okamoto M, Sakiyama J, Kurazono S, Mori S, Nakata Y, Nakaya N, et al. Developmentally regulated expression of brain-specific chondroitin sulfate proteoglycans, neurocan and phosphacan, in the postnatal rat hippocampus. Cell and Tissue Research. 2001;**306**(2):217-229. DOI: 10.1007/s004410100441

[232] Kurazono S, Okamoto M, Sakiyama J, Mori S, Nakata Y, Fukuoka J, et al. Expression of brain specific chondroitin sulfate proteoglycans, neurocan and phosphacan, in the developing and adult hippocampus of Ihara's epileptic rats. Brain Research. 2001;**898**(1):36-48. DOI: 10.1016/s0006-8993(01)02128-x

[233] Matsui F, Kawashima S, Shuo T, Yamauchi S, Tokita Y, Aono S, et al. Transient expression of juvenile-type neurocan by reactive astrocytes in adult rat brains injured by kainate-induced seizures as well as surgical incision. Neuroscience. 2002;**112**(4):773-781. DOI: 10.1016/s0306-4522(02)00136-7

[234] Heck N, Garwood J, Loeffler JP, Larmet Y, Faissner A. Differential upregulation of extracellular matrix molecules associated with the appearance of granule cell dispersion and mossy fiber sprouting during epileptogenesis in a murine model of temporal lobe epilepsy. Neuroscience. 2004;**129**(2):309-324. DOI: 10.1016/j.neuroscience.2004.06.078

[235] Okamoto M, Sakiyama J, Mori S, Kurazono S, Usui S, Hasegawa M, et al. Kainic acid-induced convulsions cause prolonged changes in the

chondroitin sulfate proteoglycans neurocan and phosphacan in the limbic structures. Experimental Neurology. 2003;**184**(1):179-195. DOI: 10.1016/s0014-4886(03)00251-6

[236] Dazzo E, Nobile C. Epilepsy-causing Reelin mutations result in impaired secretion and intracellular degradation of mutant proteins. Human Molecular Genetics. 2022;**31**(5):665-673. DOI: 10.1093/hmg/ddab271

[237] Limanaqi F, Biagioni F, Busceti CL, Ryskalin L, Soldani P, Frati A, et al. Cell clearing systems bridging neuro-immunity and synaptic plasticity. International Journal of Molecular Sciences. 2019;**20**(9):2197. DOI: 10.3390/ijms20092197

[238] Limanaqi F, Biagioni F, Busceti CL, Fabrizi C, Frati A, Fornai F. mTOR-related cell-clearing Systems in Epileptic Seizures, an update. International Journal of Molecular Sciences. 2020;**21**(5):1642. DOI: 10.3390/ijms21051642

[239] Zhu H, Wang W, Li Y. Molecular mechanism and regulation of autophagy and its potential role in epilepsy. Cells. 2022;**11**(17):2621. DOI: 10.3390/cells11172621

[240] Beck H, Goussakov IV, Lie A, Helmstaedter C, Elger CE. Synaptic plasticity in the human dentate gyrus. The Journal of Neuroscience. 2000;**20**(18):7080-7086. DOI: 10.1523/JNEUROSCI.20-18-07080.2000

[241] Leung LS, Wu C. Kindling suppresses primed-burst-induced long-term potentiation in hippocampal CA1. Neuroreport. 2003;**14**(2):211-214. DOI: 10.1097/00001756-200302100-00010

[242] Hu B, Karnup S, Zhou L, Stelzer A. Reversal of hippocampal LTP by spontaneous seizure-like activity: Role of group I mGluR and cell depolarization. Journal of Neurophysiology. 2005;**93**(1):316-336. DOI: 10.1152/jn.00172.2004

[243] Esmaeilpour K, Sheibani V, Shabani M, Mirnajafi-Zadeh J. Effect of low frequency electrical stimulation on seizure-induced short- and long-term impairments in learning and memory in rats. Physiology & Behavior. 2017;**168**:112-121. DOI: 10.1016/j.physbeh.2016.11.001

[244] Bonansco C, Couve A, Perea G, Ferradas CÁ, Roncagliolo M, Fuenzalida M. Glutamate released spontaneously from astrocytes sets the threshold for synaptic plasticity. The European Journal of Neuroscience. 2011;**33**(8):1483-1492. DOI: 10.1111/j.1460-9568.2011.07631.x

[245] Perea G, Araque A. Properties of synaptically evoked astrocyte calcium signal reveal synaptic information processing by astrocytes. Journal of Neuroscience. 2005;**25**(9):2192-2203. DOI: 10.1523/JNEUROSCI.3965-04.2005. Erratum in: The Journal of Neuroscience 2005 Mar 16;25(11):3022

[246] Perea G, Araque A. Astrocytes potentiate transmitter release at single hippocampal synapses. Science. 2007;**317**(5841):1083-1086. DOI: 10.1126/science.1144640

[247] Martorell A, Wellmann M, Guiffa F, Fuenzalida M, Bonansco C. P2Y1 receptor inhibition rescues impaired synaptic plasticity and astroglial Ca^{2+}-dependent activity in the epileptic hippocampus. Neurobiology of Disease. 2020;**146**:105132. DOI: 10.1016/j.nbd.2020.105132

[248] Parsons CG, Danysz W, Quack G. Memantine is a clinically well tolerated N-methyl-D-aspartate (NMDA) receptor

antagonist–a review of preclinical data. Neuropharmacology. 1999;**38**(6):735-767. DOI: 10.1016/s0028-3908(99)00019-2

[249] Kishi T, Matsunaga S, Oya K, Nomura I, Ikuta T, Iwata N. Memantine for Alzheimer's disease: An updated systematic review and meta-analysis. Journal of Alzheimer's Disease. 2017;**60**(2):401-425

[250] Matsunaga S, Kishi T, Nomura I, Sakuma K, Okuya M, Ikuta T, et al. The efficacy and safety of memantine for the treatment of Alzheimer's disease. Expert Opinion on Drug Safety. 2018;**17**(10):1053-1061. DOI: 10.1080/14740338.2018.1524870

[251] Vestring S, Dorner A, Scholliers J, Ehrenberger K, Kiss A, Arenz L, et al. D-Cycloserine enhances the bidirectional range of NMDAR-dependent hippocampal synaptic plasticity. Translational Psychiatry. 2024;**14**(1):18. DOI: 10.1038/s41398-023-02725-7

[252] Goff DC. D-cycloserine in schizophrenia: New strategies for improving clinical outcomes by enhancing plasticity. Current Neuropharmacology. 2017;**15**(1): 21-34. DOI: 10.2174/1570159x146661602 25154812

[253] Lynch G, Gall CM. Ampakines and the threefold path to cognitive enhancement. Trends in Neurosciences. 2006;**29**(10):554-562. DOI: 10.1016/j. tins.2006.07.007

[254] Arai AC, Kessler M. Pharmacology of ampakine modulators: From AMPA receptors to synapses and behavior. Current Drug Targets. 2007;**8**(5):583-602. DOI: 10.2174/138945007780618490

[255] Seese RR, Le AA, Wang K, Cox CD, Lynch G, Gall CM. A TrkB agonist and ampakine rescue synaptic plasticity and multiple forms of memory in a mouse model of intellectual disability. Neurobiology of Disease. 2020;**134**:104604. DOI: 10.1016/j. nbd.2019.104604

[256] Patterson SL, Grover LM, Schwartzkroin PA, Bothwell M. Neurotrophin expression in rat hippocampal slices: A stimulus paradigm inducing LTP in CA1 evokes increases in BDNF and NT-3 mRNAs. Neuron. 1992;**9**(6):1081-1088. DOI: 10.1016/0896-6273(92)90067-n

[257] Leal G, Afonso PM, Salazar IL, Duarte CB. Regulation of hippocampal synaptic plasticity by BDNF. Brain Research. 2015;**1621**:82-101. DOI: 10.1016/j.brainres.2014.10.019

[258] Kline DD, Ogier M, Kunze DL, Katz DM. Exogenous brain-derived neurotrophic factor rescues synaptic dysfunction in Mecp2-null mice. The Journal of Neuroscience. 2010;**30**(15):5303-5310. DOI: 10.1523/ JNEUROSCI.5503-09.2010

[259] Marvanová M, Lakso M, Pirhonen J, Nawa H, Wong G, Castrén E. The neuroprotective agent memantine induces brain-derived neurotrophic factor and trkB receptor expression in rat brain. Molecular and Cellular Neurosciences. 2001;**18**(3):247-258. DOI: 10.1006/mcne.2001.1027

[260] Lauterborn JC, Pineda E, Chen LY, Ramirez EA, Lynch G, Gall CM. Ampakines cause sustained increases in brain-derived neurotrophic factor signaling at excitatory synapses without changes in AMPA receptor subunit expression. Neuroscience. 2009;**159**(1):283-295. DOI: 10.1016/j. neuroscience.2008.12.018

[261] Hashimoto R, Takei N, Shimazu K, Christ L, Lu B, Chuang DM. Lithium

induces brain-derived neurotrophic factor and activates TrkB in rodent cortical neurons: An essential step for neuroprotection against glutamate excitotoxicity. Neuropharmacology. 2002;**43**(7):1173-1179. DOI: 10.1016/s0028-3908(02)00217-4

[262] Yao W, Cao Q, Luo S, He L, Yang C, Chen J, et al. Microglial ERK-NRBP1-CREB-BDNF signaling in sustained antidepressant actions of (R)-ketamine. Molecular Psychiatry. 2022;**27**(3):1618-1629. DOI: 10.1038/s41380-021-01377-7. Epub 2021 Nov 24. Erratum in: Mol Psychiatry. 2022 Mar;27(3):1630. doi: 10.1038/s41380-021-01417-2

[263] Nathan PJ, Cobb SR, Lu B, Bullmore ET, Davies CH. Studying synaptic plasticity in the human brain and opportunities for drug discovery. Current Opinion in Pharmacology. 2011;**11**(5):540-548. DOI: 10.1016/j.coph.2011.06.008

[264] Bathina S, Das UN. Brain-derived neurotrophic factor and its clinical implications. Archives of Medical Science. 2015;**11**(6):1164-1178. DOI: 10.5114/aoms.2015.56342

[265] Huerta PT, Volpe BT. Transcranial magnetic stimulation, synaptic plasticity and network oscillations. Journal of Neuroengineering and Rehabilitation. 2009;**6**:7. DOI: 10.1186/1743-0003-6-7

[266] Vékony T, Németh VL, Holczer A, Kocsis K, Kincses ZT, Vécsei L, et al. Continuous theta-burst stimulation over the dorsolateral prefrontal cortex inhibits improvement on a working memory task. Scientific Reports. 2018;**8**(1):14835. DOI: 10.1038/s41598-018-33187-3

[267] Fox MD, Buckner RL, White MP, Greicius MD, Pascual-Leone A. Efficacy of transcranial magnetic stimulation targets for depression is related to intrinsic functional connectivity with the subgenual cingulate. Biological Psychiatry. 2012;**72**(7):595-603. DOI: 10.1016/j.biopsych.2012.04.028

[268] Fox MD, Liu H, Pascual-Leone A. Identification of reproducible individualized targets for treatment of depression with TMS based on intrinsic connectivity. NeuroImage. 2013;**66**:151-160. DOI: 10.1016/j.neuroimage.2012.10.082

[269] Thickbroom GW. Transcranial magnetic stimulation and synaptic plasticity: Experimental framework and human models. Experimental Brain Research. 2007;**180**(4):583-593. DOI: 10.1007/s00221-007-0991-3

[270] Hoffman RE, Hampson M, Wu K, Anderson AW, Gore JC, Buchanan RJ, et al. Probing the pathophysiology of auditory/verbal hallucinations by combining functional magnetic resonance imaging and transcranial magnetic stimulation. Cerebral Cortex. 2007;**17**(11):2733-2743. DOI: 10.1093/cercor/bhl183

[271] Iaccarino HF, Singer AC, Martorell AJ, Rudenko A, Gao F, Gillingham TZ, et al. Gamma frequency entrainment attenuates amyloid load and modifies microglia. Nature. 2016;**540**(7632):230-235. DOI: 10.1038/nature20587. Erratum in: Nature. 2018 Oct;562(7725):E1. doi: 10.1038/s41586-018-0351-4

[272] Martorell AJ, Paulson AL, Suk HJ, Abdurrob F, Drummond GT, Guan W, et al. Multi-sensory gamma stimulation ameliorates Alzheimer's-associated pathology and improves cognition. Cell. 2019;**177**(2):256-271.e22. DOI: 10.1016/j.cell.2019.02.014

[273] Spencer KM, Nestor PG, Niznikiewicz MA, Salisbury DF,

Shenton ME, McCarley RW. Abnormal neural synchrony in schizophrenia. The Journal of Neuroscience. 2003;**23**(19):7407-7411. DOI: 10.1523/JNEUROSCI.23-19-07407.2003

[274] Ford JM, Roach BJ, Faustman WO, Mathalon DH. Out-of-synch and out-of-sorts: Dysfunction of motor-sensory communication in schizophrenia. Biological Psychiatry. 2008;**63**(8):736-743. DOI: 10.1016/j.biopsych.2007.09.013

[275] Hirano S, Hirano Y, Maekawa T, Obayashi C, Oribe N, Kuroki T, et al. Abnormal neural oscillatory activity to speech sounds in schizophrenia: A magnetoencephalography study. The Journal of Neuroscience. 2008;**28**(19):4897-4903. DOI: 10.1523/JNEUROSCI.5031-07.2008

[276] Haenschel C, Bittner RA, Waltz J, Haertling F, Wibral M, Singer W, et al. Cortical oscillatory activity is critical for working memory as revealed by deficits in early-onset schizophrenia. The Journal of Neuroscience. 2009;**29**(30):9481-9489. DOI: 10.1523/JNEUROSCI.1428-09.2009

[277] Minzenberg MJ, Firl AJ, Yoon JH, Gomes GC, Reinking C, Carter CS. Gamma oscillatory power is impaired during cognitive control independent of medication status in first-episode schizophrenia. Neuropsychopharmacology. 2010;**35**(13):2590-2599. DOI: 10.1038/npp.2010.150

[278] Shin YW, O'Donnell BF, Youn S, Kwon JS. Gamma oscillation in schizophrenia. Psychiatry Investigation. 2011;**8**(4):288-296. DOI: 10.4306/pi.2011.8.4.288

[279] Orekhova EV, Stroganova TA, Nygren G, Tsetlin MM, Posikera IN, Gillberg C, et al. Excess of high frequency electroencephalogram oscillations in boys with autism. Biological Psychiatry. 2007;**62**(9):1022-1029. DOI: 10.1016/j.biopsych.2006.12.029

[280] Sidransky E, Nalls MA, Aasly JO, Aharon-Peretz J, Annesi G, Barbosa ER, et al. Multicenter analysis of glucocerebrosidase mutations in Parkinson's disease. The New England Journal of Medicine. 2009;**361**(17):1651-1661. DOI: 10.1056/NEJMoa0901281

[281] Shalaby KE, El-Agnaf OMA. Gene-based therapeutics for Parkinson's disease. Biomedicine. 2022;**10**(8):1790. DOI: 10.3390/biomedicines10081790

[282] Vinogradov S, Fisher M, de Villers-Sidani E. Cognitive training for impaired neural systems in neuropsychiatric illness. Neuropsychopharmacology. 2012;**37**(1):43-76. DOI: 10.1038/npp.2011.251

[283] Ramsay IS, Fryer S, Roach BJ, Boos A, Fisher M, Loewy R, et al. Response to targeted cognitive training may be neuroprotective in patients with early schizophrenia. Psychiatry Research: Neuroimaging. 2021;**312**:111285. DOI: 10.1016/j.pscychresns.2021.111285

[284] Brickman AM, Buchsbaum MS, Shihabuddin L, Byne W, Newmark RE, Brand J, et al. Thalamus size and outcome in schizophrenia. Schizophrenia Research. 2004;**71**(2-3):473-484. DOI: 10.1016/j.schres.2004.03.011

[285] Cobia DJ, Smith MJ, Salinas I, Ng C, Gado M, Csernansky JG, et al. Progressive deterioration of thalamic nuclei relates to cortical network decline in schizophrenia. Schizophrenia Research. 2017;**180**:21-27. DOI: 10.1016/j.schres.2016.08.003

[286] Ramsay IS, Fryer S, Boos A, Roach BJ, Fisher M, Loewy R, et al. Response to targeted cognitive training correlates with change in thalamic volume in a randomized trial for early schizophrenia. Neuropsychopharmacology. 2018;**43**(3):590-597. DOI: 10.1038/npp.2017.213

[287] Subramaniam K, Luks TL, Garrett C, Chung C, Fisher M, Nagarajan S, et al. Intensive cognitive training in schizophrenia enhances working memory and associated prefrontal cortical efficiency in a manner that drives long-term functional gains. NeuroImage. 2014;**99**:281-292. DOI: 10.1016/j.neuroimage.2014.05.057

[288] Neeper SA, Gómez-Pinilla F, Choi J, Cotman C. Exercise and brain neurotrophins. Nature. 1995;**373**(6510):109. DOI: 10.1038/373109a0

[289] El Hayek L, Khalifeh M, Zibara V, Abi Assaad R, Emmanuel N, Karnib N, et al. Lactate mediates the effects of exercise on learning and memory through SIRT1-dependent activation of hippocampal brain-derived neurotrophic factor (BDNF). The Journal of Neuroscience. 2019;**39**(13):2369-2382. DOI: 10.1523/JNEUROSCI.1661-18.2019

Chapter 2

Mitochondrial Dysfunction in Alzheimer's Disease: A Comprehensive Review of Synaptopathy Mechanisms

Sehyoun Yoon

Abstract

Mitochondrial dysfunction and synaptopathy are significant aspects of Alzheimer's disease (AD) pathology. Mitochondria, essential for cellular energy production, play a crucial role in neuronal function and survival. Synaptopathy, characterized by damage or loss of synaptic function and structure, is a hallmark of neurodegenerative diseases. In AD, synapse loss occurs early and is closely correlated with cognitive decline. Recent genome-wide association studies have identified a group of risk factors for AD, and advanced protein-protein interaction network studies have provided insights into the relationship between mitochondrial dysfunction and synaptic dysfunction. This review explores the research conducted so far and proposes future directions for understanding the pathology of AD related to mitochondrial and synaptic functions.

Keywords: mitochondria, Alzheimer's disease, synaptopathy, neurodegenerative disease, tau

1. Introduction

Alzheimer's disease (AD) is a progressive condition that results in the degeneration of neurons, leading to memory loss, cognitive decline, and changes in behavior, eventually causing death. Early on, individuals may struggle to remember recently acquired information, which is one of the most recognizable symptoms. As the disease advances, long-term memory can also be impaired, causing individuals to forget names, faces, and significant life events. The disease impacts various cognitive abilities, including problem-solving, decision-making, and the capacity to carry out familiar tasks, often resulting in confusion, disorientation, and difficulties with planning or organizing. As the degeneration of neurons continues, individuals may experience mood changes, depression, anxiety, agitation, and occasionally delusions or hallucinations.

AD is associated with the accumulation of amyloid beta (Aβ) plaques between neural cells, which disrupts cell communication [1]. Recently, the FDA approved three new anti-amyloid drugs aimed at slowing cognitive decline in patients with early-stage AD by targeting the buildup of amyloid plaques in the brain, a characteristic feature of the disease [2]. Another key factor is the formation of tangles of a protein called tau inside cells, which disrupts nutrient transport and ultimately results in cell death [1].

Mitochondria are critical organelles within neurons, playing a vital role in fulfilling the high energy demands through ATP synthesis, production of reactive oxygen species (ROS), and regulation of calcium balance, all of which support proper brain function [3]. They play essential roles in synaptic transmission, plasticity, and homeostasis by providing ATP and buffering calcium [4, 5]. Mitochondrial dysfunction is believed to contribute to various key features of AD, such as the buildup of amyloid plaques, formation of tau protein tangles, oxidative stress, and neuronal cell death. Neurons, being highly specialized cells, require a continuous and substantial energy supply to sustain electrical activity, synaptic transmission, and cellular stability. The transport of mitochondria to synaptic terminals is crucial for supplying the necessary energy during neurotransmission, while their movement along the axon ensures that energy needs are fulfilled throughout the neuron [6–8]. Mitochondria undergo constant division and fusion to maintain their health and distribution within neurons, particularly at synapses where energy requirements are especially high [9]. This chapter explores the role of mitochondria in synaptic functions related to the progression of AD and examines the potential of targeting genes involved in mitochondrial dysfunction as a therapeutic strategy to slow or prevent the disease's advancement.

2. Mitochondrial dysfunction in Alzheimer's disease

Mitochondria are essential regulators of cellular energy production, crucial for the survival and function of neurons. Neurons in the brain have significant energy requirements, relying on mitochondria to produce ATP through oxidative phosphorylation. Because neurons are heavily dependent on ATP, mitochondrial dysfunction in AD can hinder their ability to meet these energy demands, resulting in an energy crisis (**Figure 1**). This ATP shortage disrupts critical neuronal processes, including maintaining membrane potential, ion gradients, and synaptic function [8, 10], which may contribute to the cognitive decline and progressive neuronal loss seen in AD.

2.1 Amyloid-β and tau

A defining feature of AD is the accumulation of Aβ plaques in the brain. Aβ disrupts mitochondrial respiration, reduces ATP production, and increases ROS generation [11]. It also impairs mitochondrial dynamics, including fission and fusion, and disrupts mitochondrial transport to synapses [12], which are critical for maintaining synaptic energy supply and communication. Furthermore, Aβ is associated with the activation of the mitochondrial permeability transition pore [13], triggering the release of apoptotic factors such as cytochrome c (**Figure 1**). Abnormal and hyperphosphorylated tau aggregates into neurofibrillary tangles, disrupting neuronal function. It has been shown that hyperphosphorylated tau interferes with mitochondrial transport along axons [14], compromising the delivery of adequate

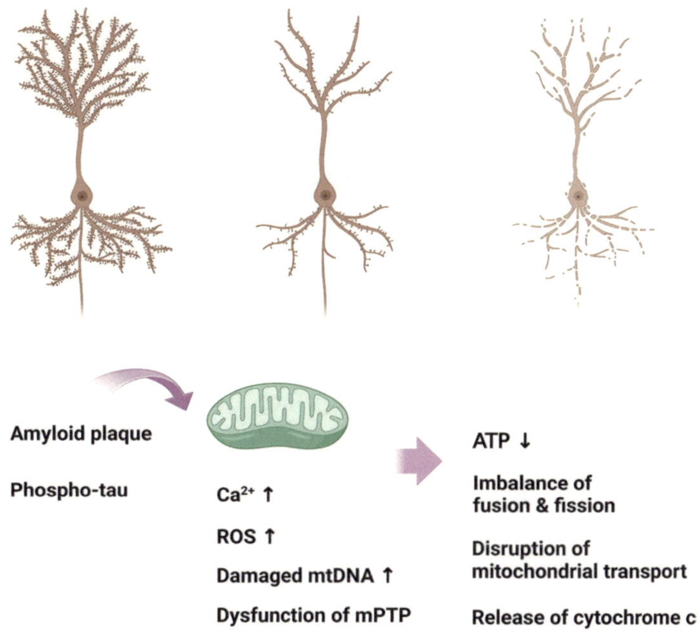

Figure 1.
Mitochondrial dysfunction in Alzheimer's disease. The schematic image illustrates how amyloid plaques or phosphorylated tau trigger neuronal cell death via mitochondrial dysfunction. ROS: reactive oxygen species; mtDNA: mitochondrial DNA; mPTP: mitochondrial permeability transition pore.

energy to synaptic terminals and thereby impairing synaptic function. Additionally, tau abnormalities affect proteins involved in mitochondrial fission, such as DNM1L, leading to mitochondrial fragmentation [15, 16]. This fragmentation exacerbates neuronal dysfunction by further diminishing the mitochondria's capacity to fulfill energy requirements. This mechanism may contribute to the neurodegeneration observed in AD by promoting neuronal cell death.

2.2 Oxidative stress and reactive oxygen species

Mitochondrial dysfunction in AD is linked to elevated production of ROS, which are natural byproducts of mitochondrial respiration. Under normal conditions, mitochondria regulate ROS levels, but in AD, this balance is disrupted. Oxidatively damaged lipids, proteins, and mitochondrial DNA (mtDNA) further impair mitochondrial function, creating a detrimental cycle [17]. Because mtDNA is located near the electron transport chain where ROS are produced, it is particularly vulnerable to oxidative damage [18]. This damage compromises the synthesis of essential proteins involved in the electron transport chain, further reducing energy production and increasing ROS levels. This escalating cycle of mitochondrial dysfunction accelerates disease progression in AD.

2.3 Calcium dysregulation

Mitochondria are essential for maintaining intracellular calcium homeostasis. When mitochondrial function is compromised, their capacity to buffer calcium is reduced, leading to calcium overload within neurons [19, 20]. This overload induces excitotoxicity, characterized by excessive activation of glutamate receptors, which causes further neuronal damage. Additionally, elevated calcium levels can contribute to neuronal death by increasing ROS production and activating apoptotic pathways.

3. Synaptopathy in Alzheimer's disease

In AD, synaptic dysfunction is an early and critical event that precedes widespread neuronal death and the cognitive decline associated with the disease. Synaptic loss is one of the most robust pathological indicators of cognitive decline in AD, with its extent closely linked to disease severity [21, 22]. This loss disrupts communication between neurons, impairing the brain's ability to process information, particularly in regions such as the hippocampus and cortex, which are crucial for memory, learning, and executive functions. The term "synaptopathy" refers to the dysfunction and degeneration of synapses—the connections through which neurons communicate. Synaptopathy manifests early in the course of AD, often occurring before significant neuronal death, indicating that synaptopathy may be a precursor to subsequent neurodegenerative events. Recognized as a primary contributor to both early and late stages of AD, synaptopathy is now a critical focus for potential therapeutic strategies aimed at preserving and restoring synaptic function.

3.1 Amyloid-β and tau

Aβ oligomers can accumulate at synapses and disrupt their function well before the formation of visible plaques [23]. These oligomers bind to synaptic receptors, including NMDA (N-methyl-D-aspartic acid) and AMPA (α-amino-3-hydroxy-5-methyl-4-isoxazolepropionic acid) receptors, which are crucial for synaptic plasticity and memory formation [24]. This interaction disrupts long-term potentiation (LTP), a key mechanism for learning and memory. Moreover, overstimulation of NMDA receptors increases susceptibility to neurotoxicity by causing excessive calcium influx, leading to neuronal damage [25]. In AD, the presence of Aβ oligomers and tau pathology can also result in excessive glutamate release, the brain's primary excitatory neurotransmitter. This chronic excitotoxicity accelerates synaptic loss, further impairing cognitive function. Abnormal tau disrupts axonal transport, which is vital for delivering synaptic proteins to synaptic terminals [14]. This disruption hinders synaptic function and contributes to synapse loss. Recent studies have also indicated that tau may have direct toxic effects on synapses. Tau can accumulate at synapses, leading to synaptic dysfunction and a decrease in synaptic density [26].

3.2 Synaptic energy deficiency

Synapses require substantial energy to support neurotransmitter release, maintain ion gradients, and facilitate synaptic plasticity. As previously discussed, mitochondria located in synaptic terminals are critical for fulfilling these energy needs. In AD, mitochondrial dysfunction reduces energy production at synapses, leading to impaired synaptic function. Without adequate energy, synapses are unable to sustain signal transmission or undergo the plastic changes necessary for memory and learning. The electron transport chain (ETC) is crucial for ATP production in mitochondria, consisting of multiple complexes that transfer electrons and create a proton gradient used by ATP synthase to generate ATP. Inefficiencies in the ETC, often caused by mitochondrial dysfunction, result in electron leakage, increased ROS production and reduced ATP synthesis [27]. Excessive ROS can damage mitochondrial proteins, lipids, and DNA, further impairing mitochondrial function and creating a cycle of increased oxidative stress and energy deficiency. This process can exacerbate synaptic dysfunction.

4. Recent findings: GWAS and PPI network studies

Genome-wide association studies (GWAS) have shed light on the genetic basis of AD. Recent findings from GWAS have identified new risk factors for AD and dementia [28], in addition to those previously reported [29]. Protein-protein interaction (PPI) networks have been employed to investigate the interplay between mitochondrial and synaptic dysfunctions, offering a systems-level perspective of AD pathology. Among the reported risk factors, three genes—BCKDK, CLU, and COX7C—were found to be directly involved in mitochondrial function (**Figure 2**; highlighted in blue). By focusing

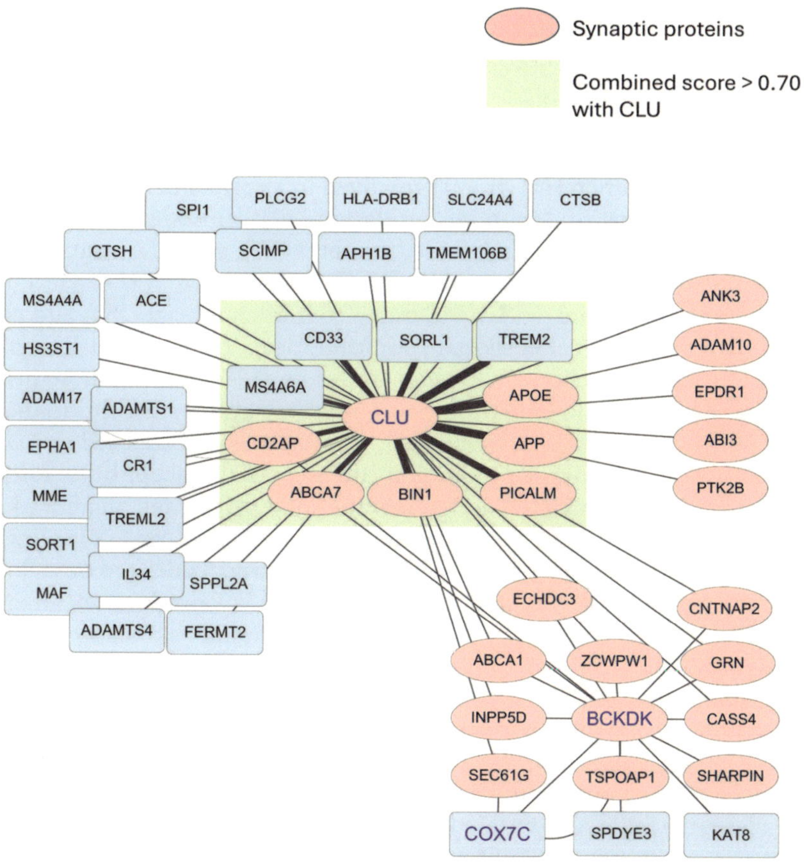

Figure 2.
Protein-protein interaction network analysis of Alzheimer's disease risk factors. Mitochondrial proteins, BCKDK, and COX7C, and mitochondrial regulatory protein, CLU, are analyzed using the STRING database and visualized with the Cytoscape program. The network depicts their relationships with other AD-related proteins. Green rectangle: combined sore over 0.700 (high confidence); Blue letters: mitochondrial and mitochondrial regulatory proteins; Pink oval: synaptic proteins.

on these three genes, the PPI network of all AD risk factors was analyzed using the STRING database (https://string-db.org), revealing 54 factors functionally related to one another (**Figure 2**). To verify the potential involvement of these 54 factors in synaptic functions, the SynGO database and synapse proteomics datasets (https://www.genes2cognition.org) were utilized for analysis. Consequently, 23 of these factors are likely to be involved in mitochondrial functions within synapses (**Figure 2**). Notably, well-studied high-risk AD genes such as apolipoprotein E (APOE) (0.999), amyloid precursor protein (APP) (0.998), bridging integrator 1 (BIN1) (0.955), and phosphatidylinositol binding clathrin assembly protein (PICALM) (0.923) were found to be expressed in synapses and highly correlated with the functional regulation of CLU.

5. Linking mitochondrial dysfunction and synaptopathy

The connection between mitochondrial dysfunction and synaptic dysfunction is a central aspect of AD pathology, with several AD risk genes localized at the synapse and involved in regulating mitochondrial function. Mitochondrial dysfunction contributes to synaptic damage, while synaptic dysfunction, in turn, worsens mitochondrial abnormalities. The role of potential risk factors that influence both of the mechanisms identified above needs to be explored.

5.1 CLU (clusterin)

Clusterin is a multifunctional protein involved in a variety of processes, including lipid transport, apoptosis, and immune regulation [30]. It also plays a role in cellular stress responses and clearance of misfolded proteins [31], and CLU mutations can impair the ability of cells to manage oxidative stress. Defective CLU can lead to excessive ROS production [32] and oxidative damage to mitochondrial DNA and proteins, which exacerbates neurodegeneration. In addition, proper mitochondrial dynamics (the balance between mitochondrial fusion and fission) is essential for maintaining a healthy mitochondrial population. Mutations in CLU can disrupt this balance, leading to mitochondrial fragmentation [33], which has been observed in AD and is associated with impaired energy production and increased susceptibility to apoptosis. Clusterin has also been implicated in the clearance of Aβ peptides, a hallmark of AD pathology [32]. Mutations in CLU can decrease the ability to clear Aβ, leading to Aβ accumulation. Aβ can directly interact with mitochondria, leading to mitochondrial dysfunction, increased ROS production, and impaired ATP production, all of which are implicated in the neurodegenerative process of Alzheimer's disease.

5.2 APOE (apolipoprotein E)

The APOE gene encodes apolipoprotein E (ApoE), a protein crucial for lipid metabolism, neuronal repair, and the clearance of Aβ [34]. ApoE plays a pivotal role in clearing Aβ peptides from the brain, preventing their toxic accumulation and the formation of amyloid plaques, a hallmark of AD. Mutations in the APOE gene can impair this clearance process, resulting in increased Aβ accumulation. In individuals carrying the APOE ε4 variant, increased production of mitochondrial ROS has been shown to cause oxidative damage to neurons [35]. This oxidative stress can damage mitochondrial DNA, lipids, and proteins, compromising mitochondrial function and contributing to neuronal death. In neurons with the APOE ε4 variant, mitochondrial dynamics, encompassing processes such as fusion and fission, are disrupted, leading to mitochondrial fragmentation and diminished energy production [35]. This dysfunction weakens the cell's ability to withstand stress and recover from damage, thereby accelerating neurodegeneration in AD. Additionally, ApoE is involved in lipid transport and homeostasis, critical for maintaining the structural integrity of cellular and mitochondrial membranes [34, 36]. The ApoE4 variant disrupts lipid metabolism, negatively impacting mitochondrial membranes and impairing their capacity to produce energy and regulate ion transport. Furthermore, mitochondrial biogenesis—the process of generating new mitochondria—is vital for sustaining cellular energy balance. The ApoE4 variant is linked to decreased expression of key regulators of mitochondrial biogenesis, such as peroxisome proliferator-activated receptor gamma coactivator 1-alpha (PGC-1α), resulting in a reduction in both the number and functionality of mitochondria [37]. This decline contributes to the energy deficits observed in AD, further perpetuating the cycle of mitochondrial dysfunction and neurodegeneration.

5.3 APP (amyloid precursor protein)

APP (amyloid precursor protein) is a membrane-embedded protein that, through specific enzymatic processing, can produce Aβ peptides, which are central to the development of AD. APP serves several functions, including roles in cell signaling and synapse formation [38]. It can be cleaved by different enzymes known as secretases. When APP is sequentially cleaved by β-secretase followed by γ-secretase, it generates Aβ peptides of varying lengths, most commonly Aβ40 and Aβ42 [39]. The amyloidogenic pathway results in the production of Aβ peptides that can aggregate and form insoluble fibrils and plaques. Notably, the accumulation of the Aβ42 variant is particularly neurotoxic, disrupting cellular processes, causing oxidative stress, and synaptic dysfunction, and ultimately leading to neuronal death [40]. This accumulation is closely associated with the pathogenesis of AD.

5.4 BIN1 (bridging integrator 1)

Mutations in the BIN1 gene (bridging integrator 1) are linked to an increased risk of late-onset AD. BIN1 is involved in clathrin-mediated endocytosis, a process critical for the cellular uptake and processing of extracellular material [41]. BIN1 also interacts with tau [42], a protein implicated in AD pathology. Mutations of BIN1 lead to increased tau accumulation and aggregation [43, 44], and dysregulation of BIN1 may exacerbate tau-related mitochondrial damage. This accumulation can lead to abnormal mitochondrial dynamics, specifically promoting excessive mitochondrial fragmentation (fission) or hindering fusion [45–47]. BIN1 plays a crucial role in processes involving the cytoskeleton and vesicle transport [48, 49], both of which are essential for mitochondrial movement. BIN1 is abundant in postsynaptic compartments, including dendritic spines, and is associated with markers like clathrin, Rab11, and Arf6, which are involved in endocytic and exocytic trafficking processes [50].

5.5 PICALM

PICALM plays a crucial role in clearing Aβ42 from the brain through its involvement in clathrin-mediated endocytosis [51, 52]. Mutations or dysfunctions in PICALM can decrease the efficiency of Aβ clearance, leading to its accumulation and subsequent localization in mitochondria, where it disrupts mitochondrial function.

Additionally, PICALM's role in cellular trafficking and membrane curvature regulation [52, 53] may influence mitochondrial dynamics. PICALM also plays a role in iron homeostasis by regulating the endocytosis of the transferrin receptor [54], which is responsible for cellular iron uptake. Iron is essential for mitochondrial function as it is a critical component of several enzymes involved in the electron transport chain. Mutations in PICALM may disrupt iron homeostasis, leading to either iron deficiency or iron overload in neurons.

6. Conclusion

Mitochondrial dysfunction and synaptopathy are pivotal elements of AD pathology. Mitochondrial dysfunction contributes to the disease by impairing energy production, increasing oxidative stress, disrupting calcium homeostasis, and activating apoptotic pathways. Moreover, interactions between mitochondria and the toxic proteins Aβ and tau, which accumulate in AD, further amplify mitochondrial damage and drive neurodegeneration. This bidirectional relationship creates a vicious cycle, wherein mitochondrial dysfunction worsens the core features of AD, accelerating cognitive decline and neuronal loss.

The interplay between mitochondrial dysfunction and synaptopathy provides a promising focus for addressing AD beyond anti-amyloid strategies. Therapeutic approaches such as targeted antioxidants for CLU mutations and interventions to restore mitochondrial dynamics could mitigate oxidative stress and prevent mitochondrial fragmentation. Similarly, modulating mitochondrial dynamics to restore the balance between fusion and fission could address mitochondrial fragmentation associated with mutations in CLU, APOE, and BIN1, ultimately preserving cellular energy production and reducing susceptibility to apoptosis. Enhancing lipid metabolism, particularly in individuals with APOE ε4 variants, could stabilize cellular and mitochondrial membranes, safeguarding synaptic communication.

Despite considerable advances in understanding these processes, many questions remain about the exact mechanisms by which mitochondrial dysfunction and synaptopathy contribute to AD pathology. Investigating the link between mitochondrial dysfunction and AD is crucial, as it offers promising avenues for unraveling disease mechanisms and developing targeted therapies. Future research should focus on elucidating these mechanisms, identifying novel therapeutic targets, and utilizing emerging analyses like PPI networks to gain deeper insights into disease progression and potential interventions.

Acknowledgements

This work was supported by an Alzheimer's Disease Research Center grant from the National Institute on Aging (AG072977). Graphical abstract was created with BioRender.

Conflict of interest

The authors declare no conflict of interest.

Notes/thanks/other declarations

Thanks to Dr. Peter Penzes (Northwestern University) for his generous support and ongoing research insights, and Dr. Changiz Geula (Northwestern University) for his guidance in understanding neurodegenerative diseases.

The author acknowledges the usage of ChatGPT 4o for language polishing of the manuscript.

Author details

Sehyoun Yoon
Department of Neuroscience, Northwestern University Feinberg School of Medicine, Chicago, IL, USA

*Address all correspondence to: sehyoun.yoon@northwestern.edu

References

[1] Rajmohan R, Reddy PH. Amyloid-beta and phosphorylated tau accumulations cause abnormalities at synapses of Alzheimer's disease neurons. Journal of Alzheimer's Disease. 2017;**57**(4):975-999

[2] Huang LK, Kuan YC, Lin HW, Hu CJ. Clinical trials of new drugs for Alzheimer disease: A 2020-2023 update. Journal of Biomedical Science. 2023;**30**(1):83

[3] Clemente-Suarez VJ, Redondo-Florez L, Beltran-Velasco AI, Ramos-Campo DJ, Belinchon-deMiguel P, Martinez-Guardado I, et al. Mitochondria and brain disease: A comprehensive review of pathological mechanisms and therapeutic opportunities. Biomedicine. 2023;**11**(9):2488

[4] Sheng ZH, Cai Q. Mitochondrial transport in neurons: Impact on synaptic homeostasis and neurodegeneration. Nature Reviews. Neuroscience. 2012;**13**(2):77-93

[5] Devine MJ, Kittler JT. Mitochondria at the neuronal presynapse in health and disease. Nature Reviews. Neuroscience. 2018;**19**(2):63-80

[6] Sheng ZH. Mitochondrial trafficking and anchoring in neurons: New insight and implications. The Journal of Cell Biology. 2014;**204**(7):1087-1098

[7] Lin MY, Sheng ZH. Regulation of mitochondrial transport in neurons. Experimental Cell Research. 2015;**334**(1):35-44

[8] Lopez-Domenech G, Kittler JT. Mitochondrial regulation of local supply of energy in neurons. Current Opinion in Neurobiology. 2023;**81**:102747

[9] Seager R, Lee L, Henley JM, Wilkinson KA. Mechanisms and roles of mitochondrial localisation and dynamics in neuronal function. Neuronal. Signals. 2020;**4**(2):NS20200008

[10] Cai Q, Tammineni P. Mitochondrial aspects of synaptic dysfunction in Alzheimer's disease. Journal of Alzheimer's Disease. 2017;**57**(4):1087-1103

[11] Misrani A, Tabassum S, Yang L. Mitochondrial dysfunction and oxidative stress in Alzheimer's disease. Frontiers in Aging Neuroscience. 2021;**13**:617588

[12] Manczak M, Calkins MJ, Reddy PH. Impaired mitochondrial dynamics and abnormal interaction of amyloid beta with mitochondrial protein Drp1 in neurons from patients with Alzheimer's disease: Implications for neuronal damage. Human Molecular Genetics. 2011;**20**(13):2495-2509

[13] Rao VK, Carlson EA, Yan SS. Mitochondrial permeability transition pore is a potential drug target for neurodegeneration. Biochimica et Biophysica Acta (BBA) - Molecular Basis of Disease. 2014;**1842**(8):1267-1272

[14] Cheng Y, Bai F. The association of tau with mitochondrial dysfunction in Alzheimer's disease. Frontiers in Neuroscience. 2018;**12**:163

[15] Kandimalla R, Reddy PH. Multiple faces of dynamin-related protein 1 and its role in Alzheimer's disease pathogenesis. Biochimica et Biophysica Acta. 2016;**1862**(4):814-828

[16] Perez MJ, Jara C, Quintanilla RA. Contribution of tau pathology to mitochondrial impairment in

neurodegeneration. Frontiers in Neuroscience. 2018;**12**:441

[17] Singh A, Kukreti R, Saso L, Kukreti S. Oxidative stress: A key modulator in neurodegenerative diseases. Molecules. 2019;**24**(8):1583

[18] Nissanka N, Moraes CT. Mitochondrial DNA damage and reactive oxygen species in neurodegenerative disease. FEBS Letters. 2018;**592**(5):728-742

[19] Norat P, Soldozy S, Sokolowski JD, Gorick CM, Kumar JS, Chae Y, et al. Mitochondrial dysfunction in neurological disorders: Exploring mitochondrial transplantation. npj Regenerative Medicine. 2020;**5**(1):22

[20] Matuz-Mares D, Gonzalez-Andrade M, Araiza-Villanueva MG, Vilchis-Landeros MM, Vazquez-Meza H. Mitochondrial calcium: Effects of its imbalance in disease. Antioxidants (Basel). 2022;**11**(5):801

[21] Subramanian J, Savage JC, Tremblay ME. Synaptic loss in Alzheimer's disease: Mechanistic insights provided by two-photon in vivo imaging of transgenic mouse models. Frontiers in Cellular Neuroscience. 2020;**14**:592607

[22] Zhang J, Wang J, Xu X, You Z, Huang Q, Huang Y, et al. In vivo synaptic density loss correlates with impaired functional and related structural connectivity in Alzheimer's disease. Journal of Cerebral Blood Flow and Metabolism. 2023;**43**(6):977-988

[23] Lacor PN, Buniel MC, Chang L, Fernandez SJ, Gong Y, Viola KL, et al. Synaptic targeting by Alzheimer's-related amyloid beta oligomers. The Journal of Neuroscience. 2004;**24**(45):10191-10200

[24] Zhang H, Jiang X, Ma L, Wei W, Li Z, Chang S, et al. Role of Abeta in Alzheimer's-related synaptic dysfunction. Frontiers in Cell and Development Biology. 2022;**10**:964075

[25] Mark LP, Prost RW, Ulmer JL, Smith MM, Daniels DL, Strottmann JM, et al. Pictorial review of glutamate excitotoxicity: Fundamental concepts for neuroimaging. AJNR. American Journal of Neuroradiology. 2001;**22**(10):1813-1824

[26] Colom-Cadena M, Davies C, Sirisi S, Lee JE, Simzer EM, Tzioras M, et al. Synaptic oligomeric tau in Alzheimer's disease—A potential culprit in the spread of tau pathology through the brain. Neuron. 2023;**111**(14):2170-83.e6

[27] Vos M, Lauwers E, Verstreken P. Synaptic mitochondria in synaptic transmission and organization of vesicle pools in health and disease. Frontiers in Synaptic Neuroscience. 2010;**2**:139

[28] Bellenguez C, Küçükali F, Jansen IE, Kleineidam L, Moreno-Grau S, Amin N, et al. New insights into the genetic etiology of Alzheimer's disease and related dementias. Nature Genetics. 2022;**54**(4):412-436

[29] Jansen IE, Savage JE, Watanabe K, Bryois J, Williams DM, Steinberg S, et al. Genome-wide meta-analysis identifies new loci and functional pathways influencing Alzheimer's disease risk. Nature Genetics. 2019;**51**(3):404-413

[30] Kovacs P, Pushparaj PN, Takacs R, Mobasheri A, Matta C. The clusterin connectome: Emerging players in chondrocyte biology and putative exploratory biomarkers of osteoarthritis. Frontiers in Immunology. 2023;**14**:1103097

[31] Satapathy S, Walker H, Brown J, Gambin Y, Wilson MR. The N-end rule pathway regulates ER stress-induced

clusterin release to the cytosol where it directs misfolded proteins for degradation. Cell Reports. 2023;**42**(9):113059

[32] Foster EM, Dangla-Valls A, Lovestone S, Ribe EM, Buckley NJ. Clusterin in Alzheimer's disease: Mechanisms, genetics, and lessons from other pathologies. Frontiers in Neuroscience. 2019;**13**:164

[33] Tang S, Ye S, Ma Y, Liang Y, Liang N, Xiao F. Clusterin alleviates Cr(VI)-induced mitochondrial apoptosis in L02 hepatocytes via inhibition of Ca(2+)-ROS-Drp1-mitochondrial fission axis. Ecotoxicology and Environmental Safety. 2020;**205**:111326

[34] Husain MA, Laurent B, Plourde M. APOE and Alzheimer's disease: From lipid transport to physiopathology and therapeutics. Frontiers in Neuroscience. 2021;**15**:630502

[35] Pires M, Rego AC. Apoe4 and Alzheimer's disease pathogenesis-mitochondrial deregulation and targeted therapeutic strategies. International Journal of Molecular Sciences. 2023;**24**(1):778

[36] Huang Y, Mahley RW. Apolipoprotein E: Structure and function in lipid metabolism, neurobiology, and Alzheimer's diseases. Neurobiology of Disease. 2014;**72 Pt A**:3-12

[37] Yin J, Nielsen M, Carcione T, Li S, Shi J. Apolipoprotein E regulates mitochondrial function through the PGC-1alpha-sirtuin 3 pathway. Aging (Albany NY). 2019;**11**(23):11148-11156

[38] Montagna E, Dorostkar MM, Herms J. The role of APP in structural spine plasticity. Frontiers in Molecular Neuroscience. 2017;**10**:136

[39] Gu L, Guo Z. Alzheimer's Abeta42 and Abeta40 peptides form interlaced amyloid fibrils. Journal of Neurochemistry. 2013;**126**(3):305-311

[40] Gouras GK, Tsai J, Naslund J, Vincent B, Edgar M, Checler F, et al. Intraneuronal Abeta42 accumulation in human brain. The American Journal of Pathology. 2000;**156**(1):15-20

[41] Miyagawa T, Ebinuma I, Morohashi Y, Hori Y, Young Chang M, Hattori H, et al. BIN1 regulates BACE1 intracellular trafficking and amyloid-beta production. Human Molecular Genetics. 2016;**25**(14):2948-2958

[42] Lasorsa A, Malki I, Cantrelle FX, Merzougui H, Boll E, Lambert JC, et al. Structural basis of tau interaction with BIN1 and regulation by tau phosphorylation. Frontiers in Molecular Neuroscience. 2018;**11**:421

[43] Calafate S, Flavin W, Verstreken P, Moechars D. Loss of Bin1 promotes the propagation of tau pathology. Cell Reports. 2016;**17**(4):931-940

[44] Terada T, Therriault J, Kang MSP, Savard M, Pascoal TA, Lussier F, et al. Mitochondrial complex I abnormalities is associated with tau and clinical symptoms in mild Alzheimer's disease. Molecular Neurodegeneration. 2021;**16**(1):28

[45] Lionello VM, Kretz C, Edelweiss E, Crucifix C, Gomez-Oca R, Messaddeq N, et al. BIN1 modulation in vivo rescues dynamin-related myopathy. Proceedings of the National Academy of Sciences of the United States of America. 2022;**119**(9):e2109576110

[46] Marmolejo-Garza A, Medeiros-Furquim T, Rao R, Eggen BJL, Boddeke E, Dolga AM. Transcriptomic and epigenomic landscapes of

Alzheimer's disease evidence mitochondrial-related pathways. Biochimica et Biophysica Acta, Molecular Cell Research. 2022;**1869**(10):119326

[47] Liao Z, Zhang Q, Ren N, Zhao H, Zheng X. Progress in mitochondrial and omics studies in Alzheimer's disease research: From molecular mechanisms to therapeutic interventions. Frontiers in Immunology. 2024;**15**:1418939

[48] Picas L, Andre-Arpin C, Comunale F, Bousquet H, Tsai FC, Rico F, et al. BIN1 regulates actin-membrane interactions during IRSp53-dependent filopodia formation. Communications Biology. 2024;**7**(1):549

[49] Drager NM, Nachman E, Winterhoff M, Bruhmann S, Shah P, Katsinelos T, et al. Bin1 directly remodels actin dynamics through its BAR domain. EMBO Reports. 2017;**18**(11):2051-2066

[50] Schurmann B, Bermingham DP, Kopeikina KJ, Myczek K, Yoon S, Horan KE, et al. A novel role for the late-onset alzheimer's disease (LOAD)-associated protein Bin1 in regulating postsynaptic trafficking and glutamatergic signaling. Molecular Psychiatry. 2020;**25**(9):2000-2016

[51] Xiao Q, Gil SC, Yan P, Wang Y, Han S, Gonzales E, et al. Role of phosphatidylinositol clathrin assembly lymphoid-myeloid leukemia (PICALM) in intracellular amyloid precursor protein (APP) processing and amyloid plaque pathogenesis. The Journal of Biological Chemistry. 2012;**287**(25):21279-21289

[52] Kanatsu K, Morohashi Y, Suzuki M, Kuroda H, Watanabe T, Tomita T, et al. Decreased CALM expression reduces Abeta42 to total Abeta ratio through clathrin-mediated endocytosis of gamma-secretase. Nature Communications. 2014;**5**:3386

[53] Thomas RS, Henson A, Gerrish A, Jones L, Williams J, Kidd EJ. Decreasing the expression of PICALM reduces endocytosis and the activity of beta-secretase: Implications for Alzheimer's disease. BMC Neuroscience. 2016;**17**(1):50

[54] Ishikawa Y, Maeda M, Pasham M, Aguet F, Tacheva-Grigorova SK, Masuda T, et al. Role of the clathrin adaptor PICALM in normal hematopoiesis and polycythemia vera pathophysiology. Haematologica. 2015;**100**(4):439-451

Section 2

Therapeutic Modulation of Plasticity

Chapter 3

The Role of Acupuncture Improving Cognitive Deficits through Regulating Neuroplasticity

Shaozhen Ji, Jiayu Duan, Mingjun Tan, Yunling Zhang and Piu Chan

Abstract

Alzheimer's disease (AD) and vascular cognitive impairment (VCI) affect millions of elderly worldwide, causing remarkable costs to society, and still lack effective treatment. Acupuncture is one of the complementary therapies that has been applied to AD and VCI, while the pathways mediating its therapeutic effects require elucidation. Neuroplasticity refers to the capacity of the nervous system to adapt to changes in internal and external environmental homeostasis, which might be the potential bridge between acupuncture and AD and VCI. This review synthesizes current evidence on acupuncture's efficacy in modulating neuroplasticity mechanisms, including neurogenesis and gliogenesis, synaptic plasticity, related regulator factors and signaling pathways, as well as brain network connectivity, aiming to establish a scientific foundation to decode the potential mechanism in regulation of neuroplasticity and optimize its clinical application as a complementary therapy for AD and VCI.

Keywords: acupuncture, Alzheimer's disease, vascular cognitive impairment, neuroplasticity, cognition

1. Introduction

Dementia is defined as a significant decline in an individual's previous level of cognition resulting in interference with their occupational, domestic, or social functioning. Dementia affects approximately 50 million individuals globally with an annual incidence of nearly 10 million [1], and is regarded as one of the most severe medical and economic challenges confronting our society. Neurodegenerative dementias are most common in the elderly [2], among which Alzheimer's disease (AD) represents the most prevalent and accounts for the majority of cases, and vascular cognitive impairment (VCI) ranks as the second contribution [3, 4]. The pathomechanisms of AD and VCI are multiple and complex, and remain limited and unknown, which include amyloid plaques and tau protein, oxidative stress, mitochondrial dysfunction, blood-brain barrier (BBB) dysfunction, inflammation, and so on [5, 6]. Therefore, there is an urgent need to explore other avenues that may expand our knowledge of the pathophysiological changes occurring in AD and VCI.

IntechOpen

Neuroplasticity encompasses the capacity of the nervous system to maintain functional adaptation to internal and external environmental changes by modifications in neural architecture, synaptic efficacy, and network connectivity [7–9], and occurs at different levels of the nervous system, from tissue to cellular to molecular [8]. Neuroplasticity takes place throughout the entire lifespan, and may be enhanced after acute and chronic brain injuries. Dysregulation or disturbance of neuroplasticity has been shown to be a pathological mechanism associated with AD [10] and VCI [11]. Neurogenesis, neuroglial crosstalk, axonal regeneration and sprouting, and synaptic plasticity are the main processes of neuroplasticity in the chronic phase of AD and VCI [12]. In addition, neuroplasticity-related regulatory factors, signaling pathways, and brain network connectivity, as part of neuroplasticity, also exert an influence on the development of AD and VCI [13]. It is therefore of great significance to gain an understanding of the treatment that stimulates or modulates neuroplasticity [1, 14, 15], and might be a potential therapy in cognitive impairments such as AD and VCI.

Acupuncture is a safe, efficient, economical and simple non-pharmacological treatment that inserts fine needles into the skin or deep tissues of specific parts (acupoints) of the body, which can be done manually, with electric stimulation, or through heating [16]. Signals of acupuncture are recognized as a potent form of sensory stimulation that ascend mainly through the spinal ventrolateral funiculus to the brain [17]. Recently, there has been a notable increase in researches to explore mechanisms of acupuncture-mediated neuroplasticity [18], which have been conducted to investigate the effects of acupuncture on the expression of genes associated with cognition and aging [19], as well as on the plasticity signaling pathways [20, 21], and functional connectivities of the brain [22].

In light of the increasing body of literature about the treatment of AD and VCI by acupuncture through neuroplasticity mechanisms, this chapter systematically reviews the application of diverse acupuncture protocols in both animal models and human subjects, evaluating their efficacy in modulating neuroplasticity across multiple domains: neurogenesis and gliogenesis, synaptic plasticity, related proteins and signaling pathways, and brain network connectivity.

2. Adult neurogenesis and gliogenesis

It has been demonstrated that the mammalian brain generates its full complement of neurons during the embryonic and perinatal stages of development [23]. This process, known as neurogenesis, involves in the generation of newborn functional neurons from precursor cells [24]. Nevertheless, a number of regions within the brain continue to produce newborn neurons and glial cells throughout the lifespan, also known as adult neurogenesis and gliogenesis, which contribute to some neurorepair and enhance brain function [25, 26]. Previous research has shown that cerebral amyloidosis associated to AD results in the inhibition of neuronal proliferation and the marked promotion of gliogenesis [27–29]. Additionally, it is suggested that stroke could induce the generation of new neurons and glial cells, particularly in the striatum and cortex [30]. Accumulating evidence indicates that adult hippocampal neurogenesis plays a role in cognitive function, and reduced neurogenesis may correlate with learning and memory disorders. In conditions where the brain is injured, like AD and VCI, compensatory neurogenesis and gliogenesis help to maintain equilibrium between the initial injury processes and the subsequent endogenous repair processes [25]. The modification of neurogenesis and gliogenesis may potentially be related to the improvement of cognitive dysfunction, and thus may represent attractive therapeutic targets for AD and VCI.

Extensive evidence established that the adult mammalian brain neurogenesis predominantly occurs in specific brain regions containing self-renewing and multipotent neural stem cells, including the hippocampus and the lateral ventricles including the subgranular zone of the hippocampus dentate gyrus and the ventricular/subventricular zone of the lateral ventricles [31]. Cognitive disorders involved in AD or ischemic injury are recognized as partly associated with the reduction in neurons, an impairment of cell proliferation, and an imbalance between the loss and proliferation of neurons in the aforementioned regions [32]. Manual acupuncture (MA) or electroacupuncture (EA) could improve the cognitive function of AD and VCI murine models by inducing the enhancement of neural stem cells (NSCs) proliferation, differentiation, and migration [33, 34]. Furthermore, neurogenesis may occur in other brain regions in pathological conditions, like the cortex [35], where the enhancement of neurogenesis correlated with EA was also observed in the AD model mice [36].

VCI is characterized by progressive white matter degeneration, featuring both axonal loss and oligodendrocyte dysfunction leading to demyelination [37]. And there is evidence to suggest that VCI is associated with adult gliogenesis, including the development of oligodendrocytes (OLs) and astrocytes [38]. As the primary cellular constituents of white matter, OLs mediate myelination that is a fundamental pathway for the appropriate propagation of action potentials along axons [39]. Myelination contributes to white matter repair in the adult brain, which may offer a promising therapeutic target for VCI [40]. In a mouse model of vascular dementia (VD), EA was demonstrated to facilitate the differentiation of oligodendrocyte precursor cells (OPCs) into mature OLs and mitigate white matter damage in the corpus callosum [41]. Moreover, astrocytes exert a pivotal influence on the promotion of neovascularization, the regulation of neuronal activity, and the sustenance of synaptogenesis and neurogenesis [39, 42]. These processes may exert a modulating effect on the recovery process following an ischemic lesion. The results of experimental studies have indicated that acupuncture can affect the proliferation and differentiation of astrocytes in VD murine models. However, the findings of these studies have been inconsistent: MA was observed to inhibit astrocyte activation and proliferation [33]; EA was demonstrated to induce the differentiation of NSCs into

Supporting facts
Increase the number of pyramidal neurons and tend to decrease the number of astrocytes in the hippocampus [33].
Promote the neurogenesis of immature granule cells and the development of neuronal dendritic spines [34].
Promote neurogenesis in the hippocampus and cortex [36].
Promote the differentiation of OPCs into OLs [41].
Increase the number of proliferative cells and differentiated cells in the hippocampus and SVZ of the ipsilateral hemisphere, and promote differentiation of proliferated cells into neurons or astrocytes [43].
Regulate the cytokine levels associated with the survival, proliferation, and differentiation of NSCs [44].
Promote the proliferation, migration, and differentiation of exogenous neural stem cells [45].

Table 1.
Potential mechanisms of acupuncture regulating adult neurogenesis and gliogenesis.

astrocytes [43]. The observed discrepancies may be attributed to the use of different acupoints or acupuncture techniques.

Beyond stimulating endogenous neurogenesis and gliogenesis, acupuncture has been demonstrated to enhance the viability, expansion, migration, and differentiation of exogenous NSCs within the hippocampal microenvironment, by modulating constituents of the cerebral microenvironment [44] or the associated cytokine levels [45] in AD mice models. The results of these studies showed the impact of acupuncture on endogenous and exogenous neurogenesis and gliogenesis in AD and VCI, which deepen our comprehension of acupuncture-induced modulation of neuroplasticity (**Table 1**).

3. Synaptic plasticity

Synapses, asymmetric intercellular junctions, are the most sensitive and plastic structures within the neuro system, and directly involved in integrating and transferring information. Previous research indicated that synaptic loss and dysfunction were a key feature in AD [46] and VCI [47], with a positive correlation with cognitive dysfunction. Synaptic dysfunction represents a pervasive initial and conspicuous pathological trait of AD, having been identified as a precursor to neuronal loss in multiple brain regions [48]. Following the onset of VCI, a breakdown in the BBB results in neuronal injury, synaptic dysfunction, loss of neuronal connectivity, and neuronal loss [49, 50]. Synaptic plasticity, the ability of synapses to modify their functional strength in response to neural activity, represents a fundamental process underlying learning and memory formation and maintenance [51]. Synaptic plasticity in the neural network represents a crucial foundation for cortical plasticity, which is linked to a range of processes, including learning, memory, sensorimotor dysfunction and recovery [51, 52]. Synaptic plasticity contains the modulation of synapse morphology, synaptic strength and transmission. These processes involve the participation of various synaptic proteins, neurotransmitters and receptors. It is currently known that modulation of synaptic plasticity emerges as a promising avenue for the treatment of AD and VCI.

It is reported that synapse-structure parameters, including synaptic curvatures, the width of the synaptic cleft, and the thickness of the postsynaptic density, serve as crucial indicators of synaptic morphological plasticity and exert a significant influence on synaptic transmission [53]. Many studies revealed that MA and EA treatments had a beneficial impact on the restoration of learning and memory capabilities in AD and VCI rats [54, 55], through the promotion of synaptic curvature, the reduction of synaptic cleft width, and the thickening of postsynaptic densities in the murine prefrontal cortex or hippocampus. Furthermore, MA was demonstrated to reverse the learning and memory impairments observed in AD model mice through the enhancement of synaptic conjunction, promotion of synaptic formation and regeneration, and an increase in the number and length of dendrites and neurite fibers [19, 56–58].

Long-term potentiation (LTP) and long-term depression (LTD) are regarded as two key elements of synaptic transmission [59]. As a physiological substrate of synaptic plasticity, LTP manifests as sustained augmentation of postsynaptic responses induced by coordinated presynaptic activity, correlating with memory formation and learning [60]. It reflects an enhancement of the synaptic strength. LTD is pertinent to the processes of memory integration, forgetting, and the restoration of LTP production in states of desaturation [61]. A substantial body of electrophysiological research indicates that acupuncture may facilitate recovery from cognitive deficits by enhancing hippocampal LTP and/or LTD [61, 62], and by preventing or restoring impaired LTP in AD or VCI models [63, 64].

Synaptophysin (SYN) is a key vesicular transmembrane protein, localized to presynaptic vesicle membranes, while postsynaptic density 95 (PSD-95) and growth-associated protein 43 (GAP-43) are postsynaptic markers [65]. They serve as critical molecular indicators of synaptic remodeling, and are extensively present in all nerve terminals and employed for the quantification of axon terminal number, indicating the occurrence, density, and strength of synapses [55, 66]. Many available researches documented a reduction in the expression of SYN and PSD-95 in the hippocampus in AD and VCI [67, 68]. It was demonstrated that acupuncture could facilitate the rehabilitation of synapse structure damage by upregulating the expression of SYN, PSD-95, and GAP-43, which was aimed to enhance the learning and memory abilities of murine models of AD and VCI [45, 54, 69].

The previous evidence suggests acupuncture plays a role in synaptic structure and function in AD and VCI through modulating the release of the presynaptic neurotransmitter or the function of the postsynaptic receptor [63, 70, 71]. Dopamine (DA) is a principal neurotransmitter that plays a pivotal role in regulating hippocampal LTP and memory processes [72]. MA has been demonstrated to activate D1/D5 receptors, to improve cognitive function and alleviate impairments in LTP in rats with VCI [71]. It is established that the central cholinergic pathway and the norepinephrine- (NE) adrenergic receptor (AR) system play an essential role in the processes of learning acquisition and synaptic plasticity in the mammalian limbic system. It was demonstrated that MA or EA could increase the expression of cholinergic-related proteins, including choline acetyltransferase (ChAT), vesicular acetylcholine transporter (vAChT), and choline transporter 1 (ChT1) [73, 74], which induced the recovery of the entire cholinergic pathways. And MA was observed to elevate NE levels and the activation of β1-AR in the hippocampus [63]. Furthermore, γ-aminobutyric acid (GABA) is a principal inhibitory neurotransmitter in the central nervous system, and suppresses the excessive release of glutamate (Glu). GABA receptor-mediated inhibitory inputs regulate hippocampal LTP [75]. EA has been demonstrated to elevate the excitability of granule cells by reducing GABA from interneurons to enhance LTP [70].

Glu receptors (GluRs) represent the primary receptors of the postsynaptic neurotransmitter region and modulating synaptic plasticity. They are classified into two main categories: metabotropic GluRs and ionotropic GluRs. Among three types of ionotropic GluRs, the N-methyl-D-aspartate receptor (NMDAR) is the most widely distributed modulator of synaptic plasticity. It has important impacts in the induction and maintenance of LTP and LTD, which are closely related to learning and memory [76]. NMDARs are constituted by the combination of NMDAR1 subunits and at least one type of NMDAR2 subunit [77]. It has been suggested that EA may be able to reduce the deficit of LTP in VCI rat models by reversing the neurotoxic effects of NMDAR1- and transient receptor potential vanilloid subtype 1- (TRPV1-) mediated processes [78]. NMDAR2 exhibits a multitude of complex properties, with distinct electrophysiological and pharmacological characteristics conferred by different NMDAR2 subunits. These subunits couple with opposing signaling pathways and exert influences on the direction of synaptic plasticity. Notably, NMDAR2A activation has been demonstrated to promote neuronal regeneration and neuroprotection, whereas NMDAR2B has been shown to induce neurotoxicity and neuronal apoptosis [79]. A study has demonstrated that EA has the potential to improve disorders

Supporting facts
Promote the rebuilding of synaptic structure by increasing postsynaptic density and narrowing the width of the synaptic cleft [54].
Increase synaptic curvatures, decrease synaptic cleft width, and thicken postsynaptic densities [55].
Enhance synaptic connectivity and accelerate new synapse formation [19].
Improve the distribution and arrangement of nerve fibers [56].
Inhibit phosphorylation of p38 mitogen-activated protein kinase (p38MAPK) and excessive microglial (MG) activation in the hippocampus to reduce the neuroinflammatory response and neurotoxicity of Aβ and promote synaptic regeneration [57].
Inhibit the activation of the ras homolog gene family member A/rho-associated protein kinase (RhoA/ROCK) pathway, and increase the number of hippocampal neuron dendritic spines [58].
Increase the ranges of LTP and LTD [61].
Increase the hippocampal synaptic transmission efficiency and LTP [62].
Upregulate DBH expression in hippocampus [63].
Increase the levels of SYN mRNA and protein [45].
Upregulate the expression of PSD-95, SYN, and GAP-43 [69].
Prevent impairments of LTP, promote the release of dopamine and its major metabolites in the hippocampus, and decrease the expression of D1 receptors and D5 receptors in the hippocampus [71].
Restore the ChT1 and vAChT expression in the hippocampus [73].
Increase the expression of cholinergic-related proteins, such as ChAT, vAchT, and ChT1 in the basal forebrain and ChAT, m1AchR, and m2AchR in the hippocampus [74].
Elevate excitability of granule cells by decreasing GABA from interneurons, which in turn results in an increase in LTP [70].
Reduce the deficit of LTP *via* the reversal of neurotoxicity mediated by NMDAR1 and TRPV1 [78].
Reduce Ca^{2+} influx *via* inhibiting Glu neurotoxicity and downregulating NMDAR2B expression [80].

Table 2.
Potential mechanisms of acupuncture regulating synaptic plasticity.

in cognitive performance involved in ischemic injury through downregulating NMDAR2B and upregulating NMDAR2A expression [80].

The EA's regulation of synaptic plasticity may be contingent upon the stimulation parameters employed. High-frequency EA may play a more robust role on hippocampal synaptic plasticity relative to low- or medium-frequency EA in AD rat models [61]. More research is required to ascertain the optimum acupuncture parameter. **Table 2** summarizes the results of some key studies. Furthermore, in addition to the aforementioned mechanisms, numerous synaptic-related proteins and signaling pathways are indispensable for the maintenance of synaptic structural plasticity and synaptic transmission. A substantial body of research has been dedicated to the investigation of synaptic plasticity-related regulatory factors and signaling mechanisms. These will be discussed in detail in the following section.

4. Neuroplasticity-related regulatory factors and signaling pathways

The process of neuroplasticity is comprised of a multitude of intricate steps, encompassing many layers of regulation. It is constituted of both intrinsic and extrinsic mechanisms. For example, the distinct stages of adult neurogenesis are orchestrated by a multitude of coordinated cell-intrinsic programs and external signals, which include the proliferation and lineage differentiation of NSCs, the migration of neuroblasts, and the integration of newborn neurons [81]. In light of the pivotal role played by associated factors and signaling pathways in neuroplasticity, it is vital to ascertain the impact of acupuncture on these elements to gain insight into the mechanisms underlying its therapeutic efficacy in AD and VCI.

Notch signaling represents an evolutionarily conserved pathway that is critical during neuronal development and specification. Notch functions as a niche signal to regulate the proliferation of adult NSCs [82]. The regeneration of neurons from neural progenitors may be hindered by an aberrantly elevated Notch signal pathway. EA treatment has been demonstrated to suppress neuronal apoptosis and improve cognitive dysfunction in AD rat models, potentially through the downregulation of an abnormal and upregulation of the Notch signaling pathway [83]. Furthermore, EA also could improve hippocampal NSC proliferation in VCI rat models through activating the Notch signaling pathway [84].

Moreover, newly born cell survival and synaptic integration are regulated by neurotrophic factors. As one of the most widely distributed and intensively researched neurotrophic factors in the mammalian brain, the brain-derived neurotrophic factor (BDNF) protein could involve mechanisms of epigenetic regulation. BDNF protein is synthesized as pre-pro BDNF and cleaved intracellularly into a pro BDNF protein, which encompasses the prodomain and the mature BDNF domain [85]. BDNF is secreted in the pro- and mature forms, which have distinct receptors and signaling cascades, inducing opposing biological functions [86–89]. Mature BDNF activates the tropomyosin receptor kinase B (TRKB) receptor, which regulates neuronal structure and alters LTP in the hippocampus, thereby enhancing cerebroprotection [90]. Conversely, pro BDNF preferentially leads to apoptosis and LTD in the hippocampus [90]. Acupuncture could upregulate the expression of TRKB receptors in AD and VCI murine models. Furthermore, it was noted that acupuncture could influence the modulation and processing of the BDNF protein from pro-BDNF to mature BDNF [36, 91], which could eventually enhance the mRNA expression levels of mature BDNF [43, 44, 54, 73]. Acupuncture may enhance calcium/calmodulin-dependent protein kinase II/cyclic adenosine monophosphate response element binding (CaMKII/CREB) signaling [92, 93], and restore the expression of CREB mRNA [73], which influences the epigenetic regulation of gene transcription, specifically BDNF. A clinical trial demonstrated that the combination of scalp acupuncture and cognitive training was effective in enhancing cognitive function and BDNF levels in peripheral blood of patients with stroke during the recovery phase [94]. Other extrinsic factors, such as neurotrophin 3 (NT3), NT4, and NT5, have been demonstrated to play a significant role in the regulation of neuronal integration [95]. EA treatment could enhance the expression of NT4/5 and their receptor, tyrosine receptor TRKB, promote OL regeneration [41]. This has been observed in a VCI mice model, where it has been linked to improvements in cognitive function.

The pathological hallmarks of AD include the abnormal accumulation of amyloid-beta (Aβ) peptide and intracellular tau-containing neurofibrillary tangles. These processes result in the loss and morphological changes of dendritic spines, which directly lead to damage of neuronal synaptic function and neuroplasticity [96]. There is a strong correlation between these changes and cognitive decline [97]. Acupuncture could regulate neuroplasticity by directly reducing Aβ deposition, with the involvement of certain related proteins and signaling pathways in this process

[98, 99]. The phosphatidylinositol 3 kinase/protein kinase B/glycogen synthase kinase-3β (PI3K/AKT/GSK-3**β**) signaling pathway has been demonstrated to play a role in the maintenance of neuronal networks, cell survival, and longevity [100]. The phosphorylation activation of AKT can inhibit GSK-3β through the induction of its phosphorylation inactivation. GSK-3β is a serine/threonine protein kinase that plays a crucial role in the pathogenesis of AD. Hand, its hyperactivity or overexpression, is closely associated with Aβ generation, tau phosphorylation, memory impairment, and synaptic plasticity [101]. EA may facilitate the rehabilitation of synapse-structure damage and enhance neuronal survival by modulating the activation of PI3K/AKT signaling and regulating GSK-3β, thereby improving the learning and memory abilities of AD rat models [55, 69]. As a downstream target of GSK-3β, the reactivation of mammalian target of rapamycin (mTOR) restored the acidification

Supporting facts
Alleviate the apoptosis of cells resulting from Aβ infusion in the hippocampus, promote the expression of synapsin-1 and SYN, and downregulate the level of Notch1 and Hes1 mRNA in the hippocampus [83].
Activate the crucial signaling molecules in the Notch signaling pathway, increase the secretion of BDNF, and promote the proliferation of hippocampal NSCs [84].
Attenuate Aβ deposits and upregulate BDNF expression [36].
Upregulate the expression of tissue plasminogen activator (tPA) protein and promote the transformation of pro-BDNF to mature BDNF [91].
Upregulate mRNA expression of BDNF and vascular endothelial growth factor (VEGF) [43].
Upregulate the basic fibroblast growth factor (bFGF), epidermal growth factor (EGF), and BDNF expression, and increase the count of neuron-specific nuclear protein (NeuN)- and glial fibrillary acidic protein (GFAP)-positive cells [44].
Promote the expression of BDNF and SYN [54].
Restore the BDNF and CREB mRNA expression [73].
Stimulate the olfactory nerve and activate the BDNF/CREB and PI3K/AKT/mTOR signaling pathways [92].
Regulate the calcium-voltage gated channel subunit alpha 1B (CACNA1B)-CaM-CaMKII-CREB axis [93].
Improve BDNF and nerve growth factor (NGF) levels in peripheral blood [94].
Mediate positive changes in the expression of NT4/5 and its receptor TRKB [41].
Alleviate neuroinflammation, reduce the ultrastructural degradation of synapses *via* the upregulation of SYN and PSD-95 protein, and decrease MG-mediated Aβ deposition [98].
Enhance the level of glucose metabolism in the brain, and the concentration of Aβ amyloid in the cortex [99].
Downregulate the expression of GSK-3β, amyloid precursor protein, and Aβ 1–40 [55].
Enhance the level of PI3K/AKT signaling, and inhibit the phosphorylation of GSK-3β [69].
Reduce BACE1 deposition and regulate PKA and LTP [64].
Promote LTP and upregulate expression of p70S6 kinase and ribosomal protein S6 in the hippocampus [105].
Upregulate expression of mTOR and eukaryotic translation initiation factor 4E (eIF4E) in the hippocampus [106].
Upregulate YB-1 expression [19].
Increase the expression of SYN and PSD-95, and inhibit AMPK activation and eEF2K activity [107].

Table 3.
Potential mechanisms of acupuncture regulating neuroplasticity-related regulatory factors and signaling pathways.

of the autophagy lysosome, thereby further promoting the clearance of pathological Aβ plaques [102]. One study showed that EA enhanced cognitive behavior in AD rats by activating the PI3K/AKT/mTOR signaling pathways [92]. However, another study indicated that EA may mitigate structural and functional synaptic plasticity impairments and memory deficits in AD rat models through the inactivation of GSK-3β/mTOR signaling [20]. As the results of the two studies were inconsistent, more research is needed in the future to clarify exactly how acupuncture improves cognitive function in AD rats by modulating mTOR. Furthermore, β-site amyloid precursor protein cleaving enzyme 1 (BACE1) is the primary protein implicated in Aβ peptide generation. One study demonstrated that EA could downregulate BACE1 expression in an AD mouse model [64].

There are a number of regulated factors and signaling pathways that directly contribute to modulating LTP. Protein kinase A (PKA) is a positive modulator of LTP in the hippocampus and has been shown to be essential for the efficacy of hippocampus-based memory [103]. EA has the potential to enhance PKA activation, heighten synaptic plasticity, and improve memory in an AD mice model [64]. The p70 ribosomal protein S6 (p70S6) kinase/ribosomal protein S6 signaling pathway has been demonstrated to facilitate neuronal growth and LTP [104]. EA has been shown to enhance the learning and spatial memory capabilities of rats with VCI and facilitate LTP in the hippocampus by upregulating the expression of p70S6 kinase and ribosomal protein S6 [105]. The p70S6 kinase was shown to undergo phosphorylation as a consequence of the activation of the mTOR signal pathway. Acupuncture stimulation could facilitate neuroplasticity by regulating the mTOR signal pathway in rats with AD or VCI [20, 106]. Moreover, acupuncture could enhance synaptic function and reverse the learning and memory impairments in AD models through some regulated factors and signaling pathways indirectly, such as the eukaryotic Y-box-binding protein 1 [19] and the adenosine 5′-monophosphate-activated protein kinase/eukaryotic elongation factor-2 kinase/eukaryotic elongation factor-2 (AMPK/eEF2K/eEF2) pathway [107]. **Table 3** presents a summary of the findings from several pivotal studies.

In addition to the aforementioned factors and signaling pathways, other mechanisms, including inflammatory responses, oxidative stress, and glucose metabolism, were identified as playing an important role in acupuncture-based treatments for AD or VCI and in modulating neuroplasticity [108]. These molecular mechanisms lend support to the view that acupuncture may offer a promising avenue for the treatment of cognitive dysfunction in patients with AD or VCI.

5. Brain network connectivity

Neuropathological alterations and/or structural-functional reorganization in AD and VCI result in altered patterns of brain network connectivity [109]. For instance, some rapidly and reversibly increased or decreased strengths of brain network connections, also characterized by altered recruitments of functional connections normally perform a given task or the recruitment of additional network connections through not typically activation by healthy individuals. The alteration of network connectivity represents a form of neuroplasticity that may indicate the engagement of compensatory mechanisms to maintain a normal level of cognitive function or to facilitate the recovery from cognitive disorders resulting from primary white matter lesions and neuronal loss [110].

Supporting facts
Modulate default mode network (DMN) activity, with increased cluster in the left posterior cingulate cortex (PCC), the right middle temporal gyrus (MTG), together with the right inferior parietal lobule (IPL), and decreased bilateral cingulate gyrus (CG) and left PCu within DMN connectivity [22].
Induce right main hemisphere activations (temporal lobe, e.g., hippocampal gyrus, insula, and some areas of the parietal lobe) and left activated regions (temporal lobe, parietal lobule, and some regions of the cerebellum) [112].
Increase the functional connectivity between the posterior cingulate gyrus (PCG)-left middle frontal gyrus (MFG) and the PCG-right superior temporal gyrus (STG) [113].

Table 4.
Potential mechanisms of acupuncture regulating brain network connectivity.

Some neuroimaging studies have indicated that acupuncture may induce neuroplastic reorganization of brain functional networks in individuals diagnosed with AD [111]. A number of regions exhibited increased or decreased activity in AD patients following MA or EA, including those related to cognition, emotion, sensorimotor function, vision, the basal ganglia, and the cerebellum [22, 112]. Further research has indicated that the impact of acupuncture on brain network connectivity in AD may be associated with a number of factors, including the specific acupoints used, the depth of stimulation, and the frequency of EA treatment. The application of different single acupoints or a combination of acupoints may result in the activation of distinct brain regions, thereby influencing the overall therapeutic efficacy of acupuncture [111]. It is hypothesized that deep stimulation at appropriate acupoints may result in stronger or more extensive effective connectivity related to the therapeutic effect, in comparison

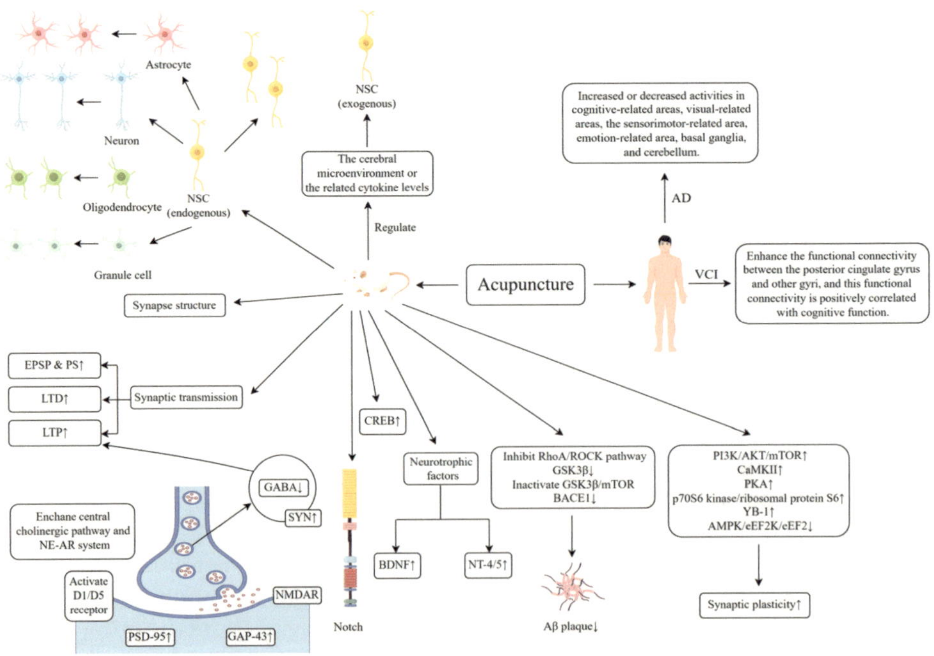

Figure 1.
Mechanisms of acupuncture regulating neuroplasticity to improve cognitive function.

to superficial stimulation. High-frequency EA may elicit a more precise brain response or reinforce the functional connectivity of brain networks correlated with memory and cognition. Moreover, a functional magnetic resonance imaging study has demonstrated that EA enhances the functional connectivity between the posterior cingulate gyrus and other gyri in patients with VCI. This functional connectivity is positively correlated with cognitive function (**Table 4**) [113].

6. Conclusion

A growing body of evidence from recent studies has gradually validated the use of acupuncture in the treatment of AD and VCI. The mechanisms by which acupuncture treats AD and VCI by improving neuroplasticity are very diverse, including the generation and development of neurons and glial cells, structural and functional plasticity of synapses, a variety of factors and pathways associated with neuroplasticity, and functional network connectivity (**Figure 1**). Given the efficacy of acupuncture in promoting therapeutic outcomes and regulating neuroplasticity, there is a potential for developing acupuncture as a promising therapeutic approach for AD and VCI.

Funding

This study was supported by the National High Level Chinese Medicine Hospital Clinical Research Funding.

Author details

Shaozhen Ji[1*], Jiayu Duan[1], Mingjun Tan[2], Yunling Zhang[3] and Piu Chan[4*]

1 Department of Neurology, Dongfang Hospital, Beijing University of Chinese Medicine, Beijing, China

2 Department of Integrated Chinese and Western Medicine, Ordos Second People's Hospital, Ordos, China

3 Department of Neurology, Xiyuan Hospital, China Academy of Chinese Medical Sciences, Beijing, China

4 National Clinical Research Center for Geriatric Disorders, Xuanwu Hospital of Capital Medical University, Beijing, China

*Address all correspondence to: jsz.929@163.com and pbchan@hotmail.com

References

[1] Zhang H, Hardie L, Bawajeeh AO, Cade J. Meat consumption, cognitive function and disorders: A systematic review with narrative synthesis and meta-analysis. Nutrients. 2020;**12**(5):1528. DOI: 10.3390/nu12051528

[2] Gale SA, Acar D, Daffner KR. Dementia. The American Journal of Medicine. 2018;**131**(10):1161-1169. DOI: 10.1016/j.amjmed.2018.01.022

[3] Scheltens P, De Strooper B, Kivipelto M, et al. Alzheimer's disease. Lancet. 2021;**397**(10284):1577-1590. DOI: 10.1016/s0140-6736(20)32205-4

[4] Rundek T, Tolea M, Ariko T, Fagerli EA, Camargo CJ. Vascular cognitive impairment (VCI). Neurotherapeutics. 2022;**19**(1):68-88. DOI: 10.1007/s13311-021-01170-y

[5] Fratiglioni L, Marseglia A, Dekhtyar S. Ageing without dementia: Can stimulating psychosocial and lifestyle experiences make a difference? Lancet Neurology. 2020;**19**(6):533-543. DOI: 10.1016/s1474-4422(20)30039-9

[6] Twarowski B, Herbet M. Inflammatory processes in Alzheimer's disease-Pathomechanism, diagnosis and treatment: A review. International Journal of Molecular Sciences. 2023;**24**(7):6518. DOI: 10.3390/ijms24076518

[7] Sweatt JD. Neural plasticity and behavior—Sixty years of conceptual advances. Journal of Neurochemistry. 2016;**139**(Suppl. 2):179-199. DOI: 10.1111/jnc.13580

[8] von Bernhardi R, Bernhardi LE, Eugenín J. What is neural plasticity? Advances in Experimental Medicine and Biology. 2017;**1015**:1-15. DOI: 10.1007/978-3-319-62817-2_1

[9] de Oliveira RMW. Neuroplasticity. Journal of Chemical Neuroanatomy. 2020;**108**:101822. DOI: 10.1016/j.jchemneu.2020.101822

[10] Jackson J, Jambrina E, Li J, et al. Targeting the synapse in Alzheimer's disease. Frontiers in Neuroscience. 2019;**13**:735. DOI: 10.3389/fnins.2019.00735

[11] Kandasamy M, Anusuyadevi M, Aigner KM, et al. TGF-β signaling: A therapeutic target to reinstate regenerative plasticity in vascular dementia? Aging and Disease. 2020;**11**(4):828-850. DOI: 10.14336/ad.2020.0222

[12] Skaper SD, Facci L, Zusso M, Giusti P. Synaptic plasticity, dementia and Alzheimer disease. CNS & Neurological Disorders Drug Targets. 2017;**16**(3):220-233. DOI: 10.2174/1871527316666170113120853

[13] Lecca D, Jung YJ, Scerba MT, et al. Role of chronic neuroinflammation in neuroplasticity and cognitive function: A hypothesis. Alzheimer's & Dementia. 2022;**18**(11):2327-2340. DOI: 10.1002/alz.12610

[14] Cramer SC, Sur M, Dobkin BH, et al. Harnessing neuroplasticity for clinical applications. Brain. 2011;**134**(Pt 6):1591-1609. DOI: 10.1093/brain/awr039

[15] Dayan E, Cohen LG. Neuroplasticity subserving motor skill learning. Neuron. 2011;**72**(3):443-454. DOI: 10.1016/j.neuron.2011.10.008

[16] Fei C, Xiao-Ling P, Xuan-Chao LI, Bao C, Yuan J, Peng H. Systematic review

and meta-analysis on acupuncture for Alzheimer disease in Chinese population. Journal of Nanchang University (Medical Sciences). 2014;**54**(9):58-65

[17] Zhao ZQ. Neural mechanism underlying acupuncture analgesia. Progress in Neurobiology. 2008;**85**(4):355-375. DOI: 10.1016/j.pneurobio.2008.05.004

[18] Ji S, Duan J, Hou X, et al. The role of acupuncture improving cognitive deficits due to Alzheimer's disease or vascular diseases through regulating neuroplasticity. Neural Plasticity. 2021;**2021**:8868447. DOI: 10.1155/2021/8868447

[19] Ding X, Yu J, Yu T, Fu Y, Han J. Acupuncture regulates the aging-related changes in gene profile expression of the hippocampus in senescence-accelerated mouse (SAMP10). Neuroscience Letters. 2006;**399**(1-2):11-16. DOI: 10.1016/j.neulet.2006.01.067

[20] Yu CC, Wang J, Ye SS, et al. Preventive electroacupuncture ameliorates D-galactose-induced Alzheimer's disease-like pathology and memory deficits probably via inhibition of GSK3β/mTOR signaling pathway. Evidence-Based Complementary and Alternative Medicine: eCAM. 2020;**2020**:1428752. DOI: 10.1155/2020/1428752

[21] Huang X, Huang K, Li Z, et al. Electroacupuncture improves cognitive deficits and insulin resistance in an OLETF rat model of Al/D-gal induced aging model via the PI3K/Akt signaling pathway. Brain Research. 2020;**1740**:146834. DOI: 10.1016/j.brainres.2020.146834

[22] Liang P, Wang Z, Qian T, Li K. Acupuncture stimulation of Taichong (Liv3) and Hegu (LI4) modulates the default mode network activity in Alzheimer's disease. American Journal of Alzheimer's Disease and Other Dementias. 2014;**29**(8):739-748. DOI: 10.1177/1533317514536600

[23] Ming GL, Song H. Adult neurogenesis in the mammalian central nervous system. Annual Review of Neuroscience. 2005;**28**:223-250. DOI: 10.1146/annurev.neuro.28.051804.101459

[24] Kriegstein A, Alvarez-Buylla A. The glial nature of embryonic and adult neural stem cells. Annual Review of Neuroscience. 2009;**32**:149-184. DOI: 10.1146/annurev.neuro.051508.135600

[25] Frisén J. Neurogenesis and gliogenesis in nervous system plasticity and repair. Annual Review of Cell and Developmental Biology. 2016;**32**:127-141. DOI: 10.1146/annurev-cellbio-111315-124953

[26] Culig L, Chu X, Bohr VA. Neurogenesis in aging and age-related neurodegenerative diseases. Ageing Research Reviews. 2022;**78**:101636. DOI: 10.1016/j.arr.2022.101636

[27] Bondolfi L, Calhoun M, Ermini F, et al. Amyloid-associated neuron loss and gliogenesis in the neocortex of amyloid precursor protein transgenic mice. The Journal of Neuroscience: The Official Journal of the Society for Neuroscience. 2002;**22**(2):515-522. DOI: 10.1523/jneurosci.22-02-00515.2002

[28] Verret L, Jankowsky JL, Xu GM, Borchelt DR, Rampon C. Alzheimer's-type amyloidosis in transgenic mice impairs survival of newborn neurons derived from adult hippocampal neurogenesis. The Journal of Neuroscience: The Official Journal of the Society for Neuroscience.

2007;**27**(25):6771-6780. DOI: 10.1523/jneurosci.5564-06.2007

[29] Baglietto-Vargas D, Sánchez-Mejias E, Navarro V, et al. Dual roles of Aβ in proliferative processes in an amyloidogenic model of Alzheimer's disease. Scientific Reports. 2017;**7**(1):10085. DOI: 10.1038/s41598-017-10353-7

[30] Lindvall O, Kokaia Z. Neurogenesis following stroke affecting the adult brain. Cold Spring Harbor Perspectives in Biology. 2015;**7**(11):a019034. DOI: 10.1101/cshperspect.a019034

[31] Zhao C, Deng W, Gage FH. Mechanisms and functional implications of adult neurogenesis. Cell. 2008;**132**(4):645-660. DOI: 10.1016/j.cell.2008.01.033

[32] Lazarov O, Hollands C. Hippocampal neurogenesis: Learning to remember. Progress in Neurobiology. 2016;**138-140**:1-18. DOI: 10.1016/j.pneurobio.2015.12.006

[33] Li F, Yan CQ, Lin LT, et al. Acupuncture attenuates cognitive deficits and increases pyramidal neuron number in hippocampal CA1 area of vascular dementia rats. BMC Complementary and Alternative Medicine. 2015;**15**:133. DOI: 10.1186/s12906-015-0656-x

[34] Ding Y, Li L, Wang S, et al. Electroacupuncture promotes neurogenesis in the dentate gyrus and improves pattern separation in an early Alzheimer's disease mouse model. Biological Research. 2023;**56**(1):65. DOI: 10.1186/s40659-023-00472-z

[35] Lin R, Iacovitti L. Classic and novel stem cell niches in brain homeostasis and repair. Brain Research. 2015;**1628**(Pt B):327-342. DOI: 10.1016/j.brainres.2015.04.029

[36] Li X, Guo F, Zhang Q, et al. Electroacupuncture decreases cognitive impairment and promotes neurogenesis in the APP/PS1 transgenic mice. BMC Complementary and Alternative Medicine. 2014;**14**:37. DOI: 10.1186/1472-6882-14-37

[37] Gorelick PB, Scuteri A, Black SE, et al. Vascular contributions to cognitive impairment and dementia: A statement for healthcare professionals from the american heart association/american stroke association. Stroke. 2011;**42**(9):2672-2713. DOI: 10.1161/STR.0b013e3182299496

[38] Lasky JL, Wu H. Notch signaling, brain development, and human disease. Pediatric Research. 2005;**57**(5 Pt 2):104r-109r. DOI: 10.1203/01.Pdr.0000159632.70510.3d

[39] Ibrahim AM, Pottoo FH, Dahiya ES, Khan FA, Kumar JBS. Neuron-glia interactions: Molecular basis of Alzheimer's disease and applications of neuroproteomics. The European Journal of Neuroscience. 2020;**52**(2):2931-2943. DOI: 10.1111/ejn.14838

[40] Franklin RJ, Ffrench-Constant C. Remyelination in the CNS: From biology to therapy. Nature Reviews Neuroscience. 2008;**9**(11):839-855. DOI: 10.1038/nrn2480

[41] Ahn SM, Kim YR, Kim HN, Shin YI, Shin HK, Choi BT. Electroacupuncture ameliorates memory impairments by enhancing oligodendrocyte regeneration in a mouse model of prolonged cerebral hypoperfusion. Scientific Reports. 2016;**6**:28646. DOI: 10.1038/srep28646

[42] Santello M, Toni N, Volterra A. Astrocyte function from information processing to cognition and cognitive impairment. Nature Neuroscience.

2019;**22**(2):154-166. DOI: 10.1038/s41593-018-0325-8

[43] Kim YR, Kim HN, Ahn SM, Choi YH, Shin HK, Choi BT. Electroacupuncture promotes post-stroke functional recovery via enhancing endogenous neurogenesis in mouse focal cerebral ischemia. PLoS ONE. 2014;**9**(2):e90000. DOI: 10.1371/journal.pone.0090000

[44] Zhao L, Zhou C, Li L, et al. Acupuncture improves cerebral microenvironment in mice with Alzheimer's disease treated with hippocampal neural stem cells. Molecular Neurobiology. 2017;**54**(7):5120-5130. DOI: 10.1007/s12035-016-0054-5

[45] Zhou CL, Zhao L, Shi HY, et al. Combined acupuncture and HuangDiSan treatment affects behavior and synaptophysin levels in the hippocampus of senescence-accelerated mouse prone 8 after neural stem cell transplantation. Neural Regeneration Research. 2018;**13**(3):541-548. DOI: 10.4103/1673-5374.228760

[46] Jack CR Jr, Knopman DS, Jagust WJ, et al. Hypothetical model of dynamic biomarkers of the Alzheimer's pathological cascade. Lancet Neurology. 2010;**9**(1):119-128. DOI: 10.1016/s1474-4422(09)70299-6

[47] Wang F, Cao Y, Ma L, Pei H, Rausch WD, Li H. Dysfunction of cerebrovascular endothelial cells: Prelude to vascular dementia. Frontiers in Aging Neuroscience. 2018;**10**:376. DOI: 10.3389/fnagi.2018.00376

[48] Yin Y, Gao D, Wang Y, et al. Tau accumulation induces synaptic impairment and memory deficit by calcineurin-mediated inactivation of nuclear CaMKIV/CREB signaling. Proceedings of the National Academy of Sciences of the United States of America. 2016;**113**(26):E3773-E3781. DOI: 10.1073/pnas.1604519113

[49] Ueno M, Chiba Y, Matsumoto K, et al. Blood-brain barrier damage in vascular dementia. Neuropathology: Official Journal of the Japanese Society of Neuropathology. 2016;**36**(2):115-124. DOI: 10.1111/neup.12262

[50] Wallin A, Kapaki E, Boban M, et al. Biochemical markers in vascular cognitive impairment associated with subcortical small vessel disease—A consensus report. BMC Neurology. 2017;**17**(1):102. DOI: 10.1186/s12883-017-0877-3

[51] Buffington SA, Huang W, Costa-Mattioli M. Translational control in synaptic plasticity and cognitive dysfunction. Annual Review of Neuroscience. 2014;**37**:17-38. DOI: 10.1146/annurev-neuro-071013-014100

[52] Neves G, Cooke SF, Bliss TV. Synaptic plasticity, memory and the hippocampus: A neural network approach to causality. Nature Reviews Neuroscience. 2008;**9**(1):65-75. DOI: 10.1038/nrn2303

[53] Bourne JN, Harris KM. Balancing structure and function at hippocampal dendritic spines. Annual Review of Neuroscience. 2008;**31**:47-67. DOI: 10.1146/annurev.neuro.31.060407.125646

[54] Xia WG, Zheng CJ, Zhang X, Wang J. Effects of "nourishing liver and kidney" acupuncture therapy on expression of brain derived neurotrophic factor and synaptophysin after cerebral ischemia reperfusion in rats. Journal of Huazhong University of Science and Technology. Medical Sciences. 2017;**37**(2):271-278. DOI: 10.1007/s11596-017-1727-7

[55] Yu CC, Wang Y, Shen F, et al. High-frequency (50 Hz) electroacupuncture

ameliorates cognitive impairment in rats with amyloid beta 1-42-induced Alzheimer's disease. Neural Regeneration Research. 2018;**13**(10):1833-1841. DOI: 10.4103/1673-5374.238620

[56] Liu T, Zhang XZ, Han JX, Nie K. Using bioinformatics tools to explore cellular biological mechanisms of "Triple Energizer Acupuncture Method" in treating senile dementia. Zhen Ci Yan Jiu. 2019;**44**(6):424-429. DOI: 10.13702/j.1000-0607.180412

[57] Wang Y, Wang Q, Ren B, et al. "Olfactory three-needle" enhances spatial learning and memory ability in SAMP8 mice. Behavioural Neurology. 2020;**2020**:2893289. DOI: 10.1155/2020/2893289

[58] Wang Y, Zhao L, Shi HY, Jia YJ, Kan BH. RhoA/ROCK pathway involved in effects of Sanjiao acupuncture on learning and memory and synaptic plasticity in Alzheimer's disease mice. Zhen Ci Yan Jiu. 2021;**46**(8):635-641. DOI: 10.13702/j.1000-0607.200985

[59] Hagena H, Manahan-Vaughan D. Interplay of hippocampal long-term potentiation and long-term depression in enabling memory representations. Philosophical Transactions of the Royal Society of London. Series B, Biological Sciences. 2024;**379**(1906):20230229. DOI: 10.1098/rstb.2023.0229

[60] van den Broeke EN, van Rijn CM, Biurrun Manresa JA, Andersen OK, Arendt-Nielsen L, Wilder-Smith OH. Neurophysiological correlates of nociceptive heterosynaptic long-term potentiation in humans. Journal of Neurophysiology. 2010;**103**(4):2107-2113. DOI: 10.1152/jn.00979.2009

[61] Li W, Kong LH, Wang H, et al. High-frequency electroacupuncture evidently reinforces hippocampal synaptic transmission in Alzheimer's disease rats. Neural Regeneration Research. 2016;**11**(5):801-806. DOI: 10.4103/1673-5374.182708

[62] Dai Y, Zhang Y, Yang M, et al. Electroacupuncture increases the hippocampal synaptic transmission efficiency and long-term plasticity to improve vascular cognitive impairment. Mediators of Inflammation. 2022;**2022**:5985143. DOI: 10.1155/2022/5985143

[63] Xiao LY, Wang XR, Yang JW, et al. Acupuncture prevents the impairment of hippocampal LTP through β1-AR in vascular dementia rats. Molecular Neurobiology. 2018;**55**(10):7677-7690. DOI: 10.1007/s12035-018-0943-x

[64] Tang Y, Shao S, Guo Y, et al. Electroacupuncture mitigates hippocampal cognitive impairments by reducing BACE1 deposition and activating PKA in APP/PS1 double transgenic mice. Neural Plasticity. 2019;**2019**:2823679. DOI: 10.1155/2019/2823679

[65] Greengard P, Valtorta F, Czernik AJ, Benfenati F. Synaptic vesicle phosphoproteins and regulation of synaptic function. Science. 1993;**259**(5096):780-785. DOI: 10.1126/science.8430330

[66] Citri A, Malenka RC. Synaptic plasticity: Multiple forms, functions, and mechanisms. Neuropsychopharmacology. 2008;**33**(1):18-41. DOI: 10.1038/sj.npp.1301559

[67] Martin SB, Dowling AL, Lianekhammy J, et al. Synaptophysin and synaptojanin-1 in down syndrome are differentially affected by Alzheimer's disease. Journal of Alzheimer's Disease. 2014;**42**(3):767-775. DOI: 10.3233/jad-140795

[68] Dong J, Zhao J, Lin Y, et al. Exercise improves recognition memory and synaptic plasticity in the prefrontal cortex for rats modelling vascular dementia. Neurological Research. 2018;**40**(1):68-77. DOI: 10.1080/01616412.2017.1398389

[69] Wang Y, Zheng A, Yang H, et al. "Olfactory three-needle" acupuncture enhances synaptic function in Aβ(1-42)-induced Alzheimer's disease via activating PI3K/AKT/GSK-3β signaling pathway. Journal of Integrative Neuroscience. 2021;**20**(1):55-65. DOI: 10.31083/j.jin.2021.01.224

[70] He X, Yan T, Chen R, Ran D. Acute effects of electro-acupuncture (EA) on hippocampal long term potentiation (LTP) of perforant path-dentate gyrus granule cells synapse related to memory. Acupuncture and Electro-Therapeutics Research. 2012;**37**(2-3):89-101. DOI: 10.3727/036012912x13831831256168

[71] Ye Y, Li H, Yang JW, et al. Acupuncture attenuated vascular dementia-induced hippocampal long-term potentiation impairments via activation of D1/D5 receptors. Stroke. 2017;**48**(4):1044-1051. DOI: 10.1161/strokeaha.116.014696

[72] Speranza L, di Porzio U, Viggiano D, de Donato A, Volpicelli F. Dopamine: The neuromodulator of long-term synaptic plasticity, reward and movement control. Cells. 2021;**10**(4):735. DOI: 10.3390/cells10040735

[73] Lee B, Sur B, Shim J, Hahm DH, Lee H. Acupuncture stimulation improves scopolamine-induced cognitive impairment via activation of cholinergic system and regulation of BDNF and CREB expressions in rats. BMC Complementary and Alternative Medicine. 2014;**14**:338. DOI: 10.1186/1472-6882-14-338

[74] Li J, Yang M, Dai Y, et al. Electroacupuncture regulates Rab5a-mediating NGF transduction to improve learning and memory ability in the early stage of AD mice. CNS Neuroscience and Therapeutics. 2024;**30**(5):e14743. DOI: 10.1111/cns.14743

[75] Arima-Yoshida F, Watabe AM, Manabe T. The mechanisms of the strong inhibitory modulation of long-term potentiation in the rat dentate gyrus. The European Journal of Neuroscience. 2011;**33**(9):1637-1646. DOI: 10.1111/j.1460-9568.2011.07657.x

[76] Kind PC, Neumann PE. Plasticity: Downstream of glutamate. Trends in Neurosciences. 2001;**24**(10):553-555. DOI: 10.1016/s0166-2236(00)01921-4

[77] Liu L, Wong TP, Pozza MF, et al. Role of NMDA receptor subtypes in governing the direction of hippocampal synaptic plasticity. Science. 2004;**304**(5673):1021-1024. DOI: 10.1126/science.1096615

[78] Lin YW, Hsieh CL. Electroacupuncture at Baihui acupoint (GV20) reverses behavior deficit and long-term potentiation through N-methyl-d-aspartate and transient receptor potential vanilloid subtype 1 receptors in middle cerebral artery occlusion rats. Journal of Integrative Neuroscience. 2010;**9**(3):269-282. DOI: 10.1142/s0219635210002433

[79] Bartlett TE, Bannister NJ, Collett VJ, et al. Differential roles of NR2A and NR2B-containing NMDA receptors in LTP and LTD in the CA1 region of two-week old rat hippocampus. Neuropharmacology. 2007;**52**(1):60-70. DOI: 10.1016/j.neuropharm.2006.07.013

[80] Zhang Y, Mao X, Lin R, Li Z, Lin J. Electroacupuncture ameliorates cognitive impairment through inhibition of Ca(2+)-mediated neurotoxicity in a rat model of cerebral ischaemia-reperfusion

injury. Acupuncture in Medicine: Journal of the British Medical Acupuncture Society. 2018;**36**(6):401-407. DOI: 10.1136/acupmed-2016-011353

[81] Suh H, Deng W, Gage FH. Signaling in adult neurogenesis. Annual Review of Cell and Developmental Biology. 2009;**25**:253-275. DOI: 10.1146/annurev.cellbio.042308.113256

[82] Alberi L, Hoey SE, Brai E, Scotti AL, Marathe S. Notch signaling in the brain: In good and bad times. Ageing Research Reviews. 2013;**12**(3):801-814. DOI: 10.1016/j.arr.2013.03.004

[83] Guo HD, Tian JX, Zhu J, et al. Electroacupuncture suppressed neuronal apoptosis and improved cognitive impairment in the AD model rats possibly via downregulation of notch signaling pathway. Evidence-Based Complementary and Alternative Medicine: eCAM. 2015;**2015**:393569. DOI: 10.1155/2015/393569

[84] Tao J, Chen B, Gao Y, et al. Electroacupuncture enhances hippocampal NSCs proliferation in cerebral ischemia-reperfusion injured rats via activation of notch signaling pathway. The International Journal of Neuroscience. 2014;**124**(3):204-212. DOI: 10.3109/00207454.2013.840781

[85] Colucci-D'Amato L, Speranza L, Volpicelli F. Neurotrophic factor BDNF, physiological functions and therapeutic potential in depression, neurodegeneration and brain cancer. International Journal of Molecular Sciences. 2020;**21**(20):7777. DOI: 10.3390/ijms21207777

[86] Egan MF, Kojima M, Callicott JH, et al. The BDNF val66met polymorphism affects activity-dependent secretion of BDNF and human memory and hippocampal function. Cell. 2003;**112**(2):257-269. DOI: 10.1016/s0092-8674(03)00035-7

[87] Chen ZY, Patel PD, Sant G, et al. Variant brain-derived neurotrophic factor (BDNF) (Met66) alters the intracellular trafficking and activity-dependent secretion of wild-type BDNF in neurosecretory cells and cortical neurons. The Journal of Neuroscience: The Official Journal of the Society for Neuroscience. 2004;**24**(18):4401-4411. DOI: 10.1523/jneurosci.0348-04.2004

[88] Pang PT, Teng HK, Zaitsev E, et al. Cleavage of proBDNF by tPA/plasmin is essential for long-term hippocampal plasticity. Science. 2004;**306**(5695):487-491. DOI: 10.1126/science.1100135

[89] Lu B, Pang PT, Woo NH. The yin and yang of neurotrophin action. Nature Reviews Neuroscience. 2005;**6**(8):603-614. DOI: 10.1038/nrn1726

[90] Lee R, Kermani P, Teng KK, Hempstead BL. Regulation of cell survival by secreted proneurotrophins. Science. 2001;**294**(5548):1945-1948. DOI: 10.1126/science.1065057

[91] Yu MY, Su KQ, Shen X, et al. Effect of electroacupuncture on proBDNF/mBDNF and synaptic plasticity in rats with learning and memory impairment after cerebral ischemia-reperfusion. Zhen Ci Yan Jiu. 2024;**49**(4):391-397. DOI: 10.13702/j.1000-0607.20221313

[92] Wang Y, Zheng AN, Yang H, et al. Olfactory three-needle electroacupuncture improved synaptic plasticity and gut microbiota of SAMP8 mice by stimulating olfactory nerve. Chinese Journal of Integrative Medicine. 2024;**30**(8):729-741. DOI: 10.1007/s11655-023-3614-3

[93] Han Q, Wang F. Electroacupuncture at GB20 improves cognitive ability and

synaptic plasticity via the CaM-CaMKII-CREB signaling pathway following cerebral ischemia-reperfusion injury in rats. Acupuncture in Medicine: Journal of the British Medical Acupuncture Society. 2024;**42**(1):23-31. DOI: 10.1177/09645284231202805

[94] Xiong J, Zhang Z, Ma Y, et al. The effect of combined scalp acupuncture and cognitive training in patients with stroke on cognitive and motor functions. NeuroRehabilitation. 2020;**46**(1):75-82. DOI: 10.3233/nre-192942

[95] Hesp ZC, Goldstein EZ, Miranda CJ, Kaspar BK, McTigue DM. Chronic oligodendrogenesis and remyelination after spinal cord injury in mice and rats. The Journal of Neuroscience: The Official Journal of the Society for Neuroscience. 2015;**35**(3):1274-1290. DOI: 10.1523/jneurosci.2568-14.2015

[96] Arendt T, Stieler JT, Holzer M. Tau and tauopathies. Brain Research Bulletin. 2016;**126**(Pt 3):238-292. DOI: 10.1016/j.brainresbull.2016.08.018

[97] Coleman PD, Yao PJ. Synaptic slaughter in Alzheimer's disease. Neurobiology of Aging. 2003;**24**(8):1023-1027. DOI: 10.1016/j.neurobiolaging.2003.09.001

[98] Cai M, Lee JH, Yang EJ. Electroacupuncture attenuates cognition impairment via anti-neuroinflammation in an Alzheimer's disease animal model. Journal of Neuroinflammation. 2019;**16**(1):264. DOI: 10.1186/s12974-019-1665-3

[99] Jiang J, Liu G, Shi S, Li Y, Li Z. Effects of manual acupuncture combined with donepezil in a mouse model of Alzheimer's disease. Acupuncture in Medicine: Journal of the British Medical Acupuncture Society. 2019;**37**(1):64-71. DOI: 10.1136/acupmed-2016-011310

[100] Bondy CA, Cheng CM. Signaling by insulin-like growth factor 1 in brain. European Journal of Pharmacology. 2004;**490**(1-3):25-31. DOI: 10.1016/j.ejphar.2004.02.042

[101] Reddy PH. Amyloid beta-induced glycogen synthase kinase 3β phosphorylated VDAC1 in Alzheimer's disease: Implications for synaptic dysfunction and neuronal damage. Biochimica et Biophysica Acta. 2013;**1832**(12):1913-1921. DOI: 10.1016/j.bbadis.2013.06.012

[102] Avrahami L, Farfara D, Shaham-Kol M, Vassar R, Frenkel D, Eldar-Finkelman H. Inhibition of glycogen synthase kinase-3 ameliorates β-amyloid pathology and restores lysosomal acidification and mammalian target of rapamycin activity in the Alzheimer disease mouse model: In vivo and in vitro studies. The Journal of Biological Chemistry. 2013;**288**(2):1295-1306. DOI: 10.1074/jbc.M112.409250

[103] Duffy SN, Craddock KJ, Abel T, Nguyen PV. Environmental enrichment modifies the PKA-dependence of hippocampal LTP and improves hippocampus-dependent memory. Learning & Memory (Cold Spring Harbor, NY). 2001;**8**(1):26-34. DOI: 10.1101/lm.36301

[104] Sui L, Wang J, Li BM. Role of the phosphoinositide 3-kinase-Akt-mammalian target of the rapamycin signaling pathway in long-term potentiation and trace fear conditioning memory in rat medial prefrontal cortex. Learning & Memory (Cold Spring Harbor, NY). 2008;**15**(10):762-776. DOI: 10.1101/lm.1067808

[105] Zhu Y, Wang X, Ye X, Gao C, Wang W. Effects of electroacupuncture on the expression of p70 ribosomal

protein S6 kinase and ribosomal protein S6 in the hippocampus of rats with vascular dementia. Neural Regeneration Research. 2012;**7**(3):207-211. DOI: 10.3969/j.issn.1673-5374.2012.03.009

[106] Zhu Y, Zeng Y, Wang X, Ye X. Effect of electroacupuncture on the expression of mTOR and eIF4E in hippocampus of rats with vascular dementia. Neurological Sciences. 2013;**34**(7):1093-1097. DOI: 10.1007/s10072-012-1209-4

[107] Dong W, Yang W, Li F, et al. Electroacupuncture improves synaptic function in SAMP8 mice probably via inhibition of the AMPK/eEF2K/eEF2 signaling pathway. Evidence-Based Complementary and Alternative Medicine: eCAM. 2019;**2019**:8260815. DOI: 10.1155/2019/8260815

[108] Du K, Yang S, Wang J, Zhu G. Acupuncture interventions for Alzheimer's disease and vascular cognitive disorders: A review of mechanisms. Oxidative Medicine and Cellular Longevity. 2022;**2022**:6080282. DOI: 10.1155/2022/6080282

[109] Fu Z, Caprihan A, Chen J, et al. Altered static and dynamic functional network connectivity in Alzheimer's disease and subcortical ischemic vascular disease: Shared and specific brain connectivity abnormalities. Human Brain Mapping. 2019;**40**(11):3203-3221. DOI: 10.1002/hbm.24591

[110] Stampanoni, Bassi M, Iezzi E, Gilio L, Centonze D, Buttari F. Synaptic plasticity shapes brain connectivity: Implications for network topology. International Journal of Molecular Sciences. 2019;**20**(24):6193. DOI: 10.3390/ijms20246193

[111] Yu CC, Ma CY, Wang H, et al. Effects of acupuncture on Alzheimer's disease: Evidence from neuroimaging studies. Chinese Journal of Integrative Medicine. 2019;**25**(8):631-640. DOI: 10.1007/s11655-018-2993-3

[112] Zhou Y, Jin J. Effect of acupuncture given at the HT 7, ST 36, ST 40 and KI 3 acupoints on various parts of the brains of Alzheimer's disease patients. Acupuncture and Electro-Therapeutics Research. 2008;**33**(1-2):9-17

[113] Lin R, Dai Y, Xu J, et al. Electroacupuncture improves vascular cognitive impairment no dementia: A Randomized Clinical Trial. Journal of Stroke and Cerebrovascular Diseases. 2024;**33**(8):107788. DOI: 10.1016/j.jstrokecerebrovasdis.2024.107788

Section 3

Synaptic Plasticity in Specific Systems and Conditions

Chapter 4

Substance P (SP) in the Retina

Fenglan Wang, Zhongqun Chen, Guiyu Guan and Jun Zhang

Abstract

Substance P (SP), a neuropeptide predominantly expressed in neurons of the central nervous system (CNS), including the retina, functions as a neuromodulator, and neurotransmitter. It is particularly significant in the context of neurodegenerative diseases such as Parkinson's disease (PD). Emerging evidence also highlights the critical role of SP in various retinal diseases, including vitreoretinopathy, retinal vein occlusion, retinal sympathetic inflammatory responses, and diabetic retinopathy. Understanding the distribution and function of SP in the retina is therefore essential for elucidating its roles in both normal physiology and pathological conditions. This review summarizes recent advancements in the study of SP and its receptor, with a focus on their distribution, physiological roles, and involvement in retinal pathologies.

Keywords: substance P, retina, distribution, function, disease

1. Introduction of substance P (SP)

1.1 The discovery and structure of SP

SP is a neuropeptide first discovered in 1931 by Von Euler and Gaddum, who extracted it from the brain and gut of horses [1]. The substance is purified and dried into powder form, hence the name SP [2]. SP is involved in the transmission of pain signals in the nervous system. It belongs to the tachykinin (TAC) family of peptides [3] and plays a crucial role in the perception of pain and inflammation. The TAC family also contains three other neuropeptides: neurokinin (NK) A, neuropeptide K, and neuropeptide C [4, 5].

SP is synthesized not only in the central nervous system (CNS), but also in the peripheral nervous system and various other tissues throughout the body. SP is expressed in many cells, including neurons [6], astrocytes [7], microglia [8], epithelial cells [9], and endothelial cells [10]. The widespread expression of SP suggests its involvement in both physiological and pathological conditions across different tissues and cells through the activation of multiple signaling pathways.

The SP peptide consists of 11 amino acids (RPKPQQFFGLM-NH2) and carries a net positive charge at physiological pH [11]. The positively charged residues are located on the N terminal, while the negatively charged hydrophobic residues are found on the C terminal, making SP an amphiphilic peptide. This property allows SP to interact directly with cell membrane proteins. Importantly, SP mediates its functions by interacting specifically with surface receptors, namely members of the NK family of G protein-coupled receptors (GPCRs) [12]. SP is relatively stable in plasma but has a short half-life in tissues. In tissues and blood, the half-life of SP ranges from a few seconds to tens of minutes, whereas in extracted plasma, SP remains stable for several hours [13].

1.2 The physiological and pathological processes of SP

As a neurotransmitter and neuromodulator, SP primarily functions in pain modulation and has neuroprotective effects, both of which operate through NK-1 receptor (NK-1R) [14].

SP transmit pain signals from the site of injury or inflammation to the CNS. This signaling pathway is involved in both acute and chronic pain conditions. In addition, SP plays a crucial neuroprotective role in rheumatoid arthritis (RA), with significant increases in SP levels in the synovial sac of RA patients [15]. SP is also critical in inflammatory bowel disease (IBD), where increased SP levels and upregulation of NK-1Rs have been observed in the rectum and colon, correlating closely with disease activity [16].

Beyond pain modulation and neuroprotection, SP is implicated in various physiological processes. These include the activation of microglia [17], apoptosis [18], vasodilation [19], gastrointestinal motility [16], and immune response modulation [12]. Each of these processes will be summarized here and discussed in detail in the following chapters. SP stimulates microglial activation, leading to the production of reactive oxygen species (ROS) and pro-inflammatory cytokines such as tumor necrosis factor-alpha (TNF-α) and interleukin-6 (IL-6). These effects can be partially inhibited by antagonists of SP receptors NK-1R, NK-2R, and NK-3R. In conclusion, SP triggers microglial activation and the release of pro-inflammatory factors, thereby promoting microglia-mediated brain inflammation [17].

In studies of neutrophil apoptosis, SP has been shown to delay apoptosis in the cornea of mice following bacterial infection, whereas blocking SP interaction with NK-1R promotes early apoptosis and improves disease outcomes [18]. Additionally, when SP was implanted into the avascular cornea of rabbits, significant neovascularization was observed. Selective NK-1R agonists produced similar proliferative effects, while selective NK-2R and NK-3R agonists did not have a significant impact. These results suggest that SP promotes neovascularization through NK-1R [19]. SP also exerts pro-inflammatory effects in immune and epithelial cells and is involved in inflammatory diseases of the respiratory, gastrointestinal, and musculoskeletal systems. For instance, patients with asthma exhibit an overreaction to SP and increased NK-1R expression in their bronchi [12].

1.3 The physiological and pathological processes of SP in the retina

Similar to its role in the CNS, SP influences and participates in numerous physiological and pathophysiological processes in the retina. Electrophysiological recordings indicate that SP exerts excitatory effects on retina ganglion cells (RGCs) [20, 21] and dopaminergic amacrine cells (ACs) [21] through its preferred NK-1Rs [22, 23]. Pathological studies have demonstrated that SP can inhibit early retinal inflammatory response, prevent cell death, and significantly delay the progression of retinal degeneration [24–26]. Additionally, SP has been shown to prevent N-methyl-D-aspartate (NMDA)-induced apoptosis of RGCs and vascular endothelial growth factor (VEGF)-induced endothelial barrier destruction [27]. Thus, SP plays an important role in various retinal diseases, including vitreoretinopathy (PVR) [24], retinal vein occlusion [27], retinal sympathetic inflammatory response [25], and diabetic retinopathy (DR) [26].

Ongoing research into SP continues to uncover its multifaceted roles in health and disease, making it a significant target for pharmacological interventions aimed at related conditions.

2. The distribution of SP and NK-1R

2.1 SP and NK-1R are distributed in various tissues and cells

Studies showed that SP is highly expressed in a wide range of tissues, particularly in the CNS, including the retina. SP is extensively expressed across various cell types, with notable expression in neurons [28], immune cells [12, 29], microglia [8], epithelial cells [9], and endothelial cells [30] in the CNS. Immune cells that express SP include T cells [29], macrophages [31], dendritic cells [32], and eosinophils [33]. Additionally, SP is expressed in several stem cells, progenitor cells, and immunomodulatory mesenchymal stem cells (MSCs) [34].

SP mediates its function through specific interactions with surface receptors, which are members of the GPCR family of neurokinins [12]. There are three typical types of NK receptors: NK-1R, NK-2R, and NK-3R, which are usually expressed in the same cell but with different affinities. Among these, NK-1R, which localizes in lipid raft, is the GPCR with the highest affinity for SP [35]. NK-1R has two isomers with different affinities: high-affinity NK-1R-F (full-length version of 407 residues) and low-affinity NK-1R-T (truncated 311 residues) [36].

Similar to SP, NK-1R is expressed by neurons [37], microglia, and astrocytes [38], as well as by epithelial [39], endothelial [40], smooth muscle cells [41], and fibroblasts [42]. Notably, among immune cells, NK-1R expression includes T and B lymphocytes [29], natural killer cells [43], dendritic cells [44], monocytes/macrophages [45], eosinophils, and mast cells [46].

2.2 The distribution of SP in the CNS

It is now well established that SP and NK-1R are widely distributed throughout the CNS. Since the mid-1970s, the immunoreactivity (IR) of SP has been observed in the CNS, and its distribution in the rat CNS has been extensively studied using neuroanatomy [47]. In addition, research has shown that SP is expressed in the dorsal root ganglion (DRG) but not in the ventral horn, providing evidence that SP is involved in primary sensory afferent pathways [48]. Therefore, SP exhibits an uneven distribution in the CNS [49].

The highest concentrations of SP have been found in the substantia nigra (SN), medial amygdala (MA), and the spinal cord dorsal horn (SDH) [50]. SP is present in primary sensory neurons in the brainstem, brain nucleus, and SDH [47, 51], which supports its important role as a sensory neurotransmitter in pain perception [51]. Moreover, SP is present in several other areas of the brain, including the hippocampus, cortex, basal ganglia, and hypothalamus, suggesting it may have significant effects on CNS function [52].

2.3 The distribution of SP in the retina

The distribution of SP-IR has been studied in a variety of species, including rats [53], mice [54], goldfishes [55], hamsters [56], rabbits [57], cats [58], salamanders [59], guinea pigs [60], monkeys [61], and human [62] retinas. SP expression is commonly found in ACs, displaced ACs (DACs), and some RGCs, but not in bipolar cells (BCs) and retinal pigment epithelial (RPE) cells. In the human retina, there are slightly more SP-positive DACs compared to ACs [62]. SP can excite ON, OFF, and ON-OFF RGCs in the retinas of fish, loach, and rabbits [20, 63, 64]. Studies have also shown that in human and turtle retinas, some processes from ACs are surrounded by SP-positive and SP-negative RGCs [62, 65]. In the primate retina, SP-positive ACs are wide-field cells with large somas that are normal or displaced relative to the inner plexiform layer (IPL) [66–71].

In the cat retina, SP-IR is located in two subpopulations of ACs with processes in sublayer 1 (S1) and sublayer 4 (S4) of the IPL [58]. In the primate retina, SP-IR is present in S1 and sublayer 3 (S3) [72], while in the mouse retina, most SP-IR is located in IPL layers S1, S3, and sublayer 5 (S5), with the strongest expression in the S5 layer [54].

Further analysis of synaptic circuits and the roles of input and output neurons is performed through electron microscopy (EM) and confocal microscopy [55, 60, 62, 72]. EM studies reveal that SP-positive ACs receive synaptic inputs from both ACs and BCs, though the synaptic outputs differ across species. For instance, in the guinea pig retina, the primary targets of SP-positive ACs are RGCs [60]. Conversely, in the primate retina, SP-positive ACs predominantly form synaptic connections with other ACs and BCs [72]. Further EM observations in the mouse retina indicate that SP-positive ACs primarily receive inputs from other SP-positive ACs and predominantly transmit signals to SP-negative ACs. This pattern suggests a sequential inhibition mechanism among ACs. Additionally, SP-positive ACs in the mouse retina also receive significant input from both ACs and BCs, with ACs and RGCs being the main target cells. This indicates a complex interplay of inhibitory and excitatory signals in the retinal synaptic network, with SP-positive ACs playing a critical role in modulating retinal signal processing [54]. The dendritic output of SP-IR includes bipolar axons, AC processes, and the IPL neuropil, primarily in S3 in the primate retina. SP-IR axons are distributed among somatic, axonal, normal, and ectopic cell bodies. There may also be synapses between these cells [62, 72]. The result showed that SP-positive ACs located in S3 in IPL were contacted with cone bipolar axons on the sublayer 2 (S2)/S3 boundary and glycinergic BCs on the S3 and S3-S4 boundary in the primate retina [72]. SP-positive axons are also found distributed in the S1 region, where they surround the strongly gamma-aminobutyric acid (GABA)-positive ACs. Some of these axons extend into the outer plexiform layer (OPL), while others penetrate deeply into the ganglion cell layer (GCL). In the GCL, they encircle SP-positive RGCs and then travel toward the nerve fiber layer [72].

The distribution and synaptic structure of SP-IR varied among species, indicating that the role of SP differs across species. SP-IR is essential for studying the complex structure of neurotransmitter systems. The retina, being a key organ for vision perception, serves as a significant research platform for neurodegenerative disease studies. Increasing evidence suggests that SP is involved in retinal inflammation and degeneration in mice [25, 26]. Researchers are actively exploring how retinal damage develops in disease conditions, highlighting the potential impact of SP on these processes.

2.4 The distribution of NK-1R in the CNS and retina

Specific and high-affinity binding sites for SP have been identified in the retinas of albino rabbits and rats using *in vitro* autoradiography [73]. Since NK-1R is the receptor with the highest affinity for SP, it has garnered significant attention. Due to its high expression in various cells and tissues, NK-1R mediates numerous cellular functions involving SP. NK-1R is widely expressed in the CNS, with NK-1R mRNA found in the olfactory bulb, cerebral cortex, medulla oblongata, and spinal cord of mice [74, 75].

Early studies in the human brain indicated that NK-1R was highly expressed in the locus coeruleus and ventral striatum, moderately in the cortex, hippocampus, and amygdaloid nucleus, but minimally in the cerebellum and thalamus [74]. Further studies showed that the highest NK-1R level is typically found in the caudate and putamen regions near the amygdala [76]. The interaction between SP and NK-1R is crucial for complex CNS processing [77].

Recent findings suggest that SP might not function as a classic neurotransmitter based on the expression patterns of NK-1R. There appears to be an anatomical mismatch between SP release sites and responsive cells, and many CNS SP receptors are located non-synaptically [77]. This suggests that SP may have endocrine-like properties both within and outside the CNS. The functional expression of NK-1R in various non-neuronal cells, including smooth muscle cells, fibroblasts, keratinocytes, and endothelial cells, supports this notion [78].

In mammalian retinas, NK-1R is reported to be present in a wide range of retinal cells. NK-1R localization has been observed on the GABAergic and dopaminergic ACs, DACs, and IPL, and some RGCs has been observed [79, 80]. Similar NK-1R expression has been noted in the retinas of various mammals [81, 82]. Double-labeling studies have showed that NK-1R is present in BCs and many ACs in the mouse retina [82]. Specifically, NK-1R positive BCs are classified as ON-cone BCs, differing from rod BCs and containing glycine. These BCs are nonrandomly distributed and have the highest density in the central retina [82]. Similarly, NK-1R IR was observed in a large number of ON-cone BCs and all dopaminergic ACs in the retinas of rabbits [83]. This expression pattern is similar to that observed in the rabbit retina [82, 83]. NK-1R was generally expressed in dopaminergic cells, suggesting that SP neurotransmission is a common feature among dopaminergic cells in the retinas of mice, rats, and rabbits [79, 82, 83]. Interestingly, ACs containing SP may also express NK-1 auto receptors in the mouse retina [82].

3. The colocalization of SP and other neurotransmitters

SP is an important neurotransmitter that exists extensively in the nervous system and often co-located with other neurotransmitters. This common distribution reflects the complex diversity of neurotransmitters secreted by neurons. When neurotransmitters are present in the same neuron, they may interact synergistically or regulate each other, which has a significant impact on various physiological and behavioral processes. Therefore, studying the co-distribution of SP and other neurotransmitters can enhance our understanding of the intricate structure of the neurotransmitter system and its functions in both normal and disease states. This research not only provides insights into individual signaling molecules but also contributes to a broader understanding of the overall regulatory mechanisms of the nervous system, which is crucial for developing and optimizing disease treatment strategies. The co-localization of SP with other neurotransmitters is as follows:

3.1 The colocalizations

Triple immunocytochemical studies have revealed that some terminals of the SN contain both SP and GABA, which are delivered to dopaminergic neurons [84]. In addition, retrograde labeling of RGCs in albino rats showed that about 3% of RGCs projecting to the contralateral superior colliculus exhibit SP-IR, with some also being GABA-positive [85]. The growing body of evidence suggests that SP and GABA may be involved in the transmission of retinal RGCs [86].

Further studies have demonstrated that SP is present in a subset of GABA-positive cells in the cat retina [87]. In mice, nearly all SP-positive ACs and some SP-positive RGCs were co-localized with GAD67, indicating that these cells are GABAergic. This finding has been confirmed in other species [20, 54, 59]. However, in guinea pigs, chickens, and rabbits, although SP is recognized as a neurotransmitter in RGCs, GABA is not expressed in the RGCs of these species [57, 86]. It is suggested that SP may inhibit some retinal neurons by activating GABAergic neurotransmission [20].

In addition, a study in mice revealed that some SP-positive cells were co-localized with both GABA and alpha-Synuclein (α-Syn) in ACs and RGCs. And this triple marker was identified for the first time in vertebrate retinas, with almost all SP-positive RGCs also expressing α-Syn [54]. Similarly, beta-Synuclein (β-Syn) and SP were found to share many co-localizations in the retina [54].

Studies have also shown that the IR of 5-hydroxytryptamine (5-HT), SP, and glutamate in the spinal cord of monkeys and rats is significantly co-localized around dendrites and large alpha-motoneurons. Their release from the same DRG may exert joint effects on SDH neurons [88]. However, their co-localization in the retinas of other species has been rarely studied, and SP and glutamate did not co-exist in the mouse retina [54].

3.2 The non-colocalizations

Research has demonstrated co-labeling of SP with glycinergic ACs in the salamander retina [59]. However, SP-positive ACs in the mouse retina did not co-localize with glycine transporter 1 (GlyT1), dopamine, somatostatin (SOM), or holiness acetyltransferase (ChAT) [54], suggesting a differential distribution of SP across different species' retina. Additionally, in ventral medullary neurons, types of neurochemicals—5-HT, thyrotropin-releasing hormone (TSH), and SP—have been identified [89, 90]. However, their co-localization in the retina is rarely studied.

4. The physiological effects of SP

SP neurotransmission is important for neuronal function and circuitry. As a member of the neuropeptide TAC family, SP interacts with G protein-coupled NKRs to elicit its effects. Among these receptors, NK-1R has the highest affinity with SP [91, 92]. Numerous studies have investigated the physiological functions of SP. Emerging evidence suggests that SP plays vital roles in the CNS, including synaptic transmission, neurotransmitter release, and other diverse physiological processes [21, 93].

4.1 SP modulates synaptic plasticity

Research has shown that application of SP can regulate synaptic transmission at Schaffer collateral-Cornu Ammonis1 (SC-CA1) synapses in the hippocampus of mice [94]. Specifically, SP acts on the NK-1R to enhance local inhibitory responses by affecting the release of GABA in the hippocampus [95]. This inhibition plays a vital role in facilitating neuronal circuit synchronization and adjusting both short-term and long-term synaptic plasticity [94, 95]. In addition, CA2, a small region inserted between CA1 and CA3, is innervated by SP-IR neurons from supramammillary (SuM) [96]. SP can induce a slowly developing NMDA receptor- and protein synthesis-dependent potentiation of CA2 synapse [93]. Furthermore, as one of the important neuropeptides released by striatal neurons [97], SP can also induce spontaneous neurotransmitter release and trigger calcium-dependent rapid synaptic vesicle exocytosis in these neurons *via* NK-1R [98]. Melani and colleagues have elucidated that SP selectively enhances glutamate release from dMHb neurons onto LIPN neurons in a NK-1R dependent manner [99]. Additionally, Yamaguchi and colleagues found that SP can modulate inward rectification characteristics of potassium channels in isolated cholinergic neurons from the rat nucleus basalis [100]. These electrophysiology results indicate that SP exerts neuromodulatory effects on central synaptic transmission.

4.2 SP regulates neuronal excitability

The retina, as part of the CNS, is widely distributed with SP and NK-1R [54, 79]. Similar to its effects in the CNS, SP influences various physiological processes in the retina. Research has shown that SP can regulate the activity of RGCs and ACs in the retina, with differences observed among species. Zalutsky and Miller recorded responses from a rabbit retina eyecup bathed in SP, noting that SP excited RGCs [20]. The same excitatory effect of SP on all types of RGCs (ON, OFF, and ON-OFF units) has been observed in the mudpuppy and tiger salamander retinas [63]. However, in the carp retina, SP only excites ON and ON-OFF RGCs while inhibiting OFF RGCs [101]. In addition to its excitatory effect on RGCs, SP also excites ACs. Zalutsky's and Miller's electrophysiological recordings indicated that SP also has an excitatory effect on GABAergic ACs in the rabbit retina, with some of the depolarized ACs probably being AII ACs [20]. The specific mechanism by which SP regulates neuronal excitability is the subject of various theories. It is widely believed that the retinal circuit mediates SP neurotransmission through NK-1R. SP released by SP-IR ACs acts on the NK-1R expressed in ON-type cone BCs, which may affect RGC activity [83]. Similarly, much of SP released by SP-IR ACs acts at NK-1R expressed by SP-negative AC processes [82], suggesting a network of inhibition among ACs. Additionally, some SP acts on SP-IR ACs, potentially regulating cell activity through autocrine or paracrine pathways [54, 82].

4.3 SP promotes the release of neurotransmitters

In addition to stimulating retinal neurons, SP can also promote the release of neurotransmitters. Casini et al. incubated detached rabbit retina in SP saline at various concentrations and analyzed the culture medium by high-pressure liquid chromatography (HPLC) to detect dopamine levels. They found that SP promotes dopamine release at postnatal day (PND) 35 [21]. Given the expression of NK-1R in dopaminergic ACs in the retina [83], they tested the effect of NK1-1R agonist/antagonists on dopamine release. The results showed that extracellular dopamine levels were significantly increased by NK-1R agonist and decreased by NK-1R antagonists, suggesting that SP promotes dopamine release through NK-1R [21].

4.4 SP regulates Ca^{2+} levels and currents

Moreover, SP can regulate Ca^{2+} levels and calcium current in retina cells. Casini et al. found that SP increases intracellular Ca^{2+} levels in "starburst" cells in embryonic day 30 (E30)—PND1 rabbit retinal flat mounts, as determined by calcium imaging technology [21]. This finding indicates that SP neurotransmission is likely a crucial developmental element for the maturation of retinal neurons and circuitries. Similar to its effect on dopamine release, intracellular Ca^{2+} levels were significantly increased by NK-1R agonist and reversibly inhibited by NK-1R antagonists [21]. These Ca^{2+} imaging results suggest that developing "starburst" cells transiently express functional NK-1R, which play a significant role in regulating Ca^{2+} concentrations during development, indicating that SP regulates intracellular Ca^{2+} levels in rabbit retinal "starburst" cells in an NK-1R-dependent manner [21]. Additionally, Ayoub and Matthews found SP regulates the calcium currents in retinal BCs from goldfish [102]. BCs, as interneurons that transmit visual signals from photoreceptors to ACs and RGCs, receive a large amount of synaptic feedback from ACs, some of which contain SP neuropeptides [54, 103]. Ayoub and Matthews observed that SP had a potent voltage-dependent inhibitory effect on calcium currents in these cells [102]. This suppression was attributed to the inhibition of the slowly inactivating L-type current by SP, which contrasts with the transient N-type current inhibition reported in frog sympathetic neurons [104]. Additionally, somatostatin and menaquinone present in ACs also exhibited a similar effect on calcium current [102]. However, further research is needed to determine whether this regulatory effect is mediated through NK-1R.

These findings underscore the significant role of SP in regulating synaptic transmission, highlight its synaptic plasticity properties, and confirm its involvement physiologically.

5. The protective effect of SP

The neuropeptide SP is involved in various biological processes [12], and its neuroprotective effect has attracted a lot of attention in recent years. Emerging research indicates that SP has neuroprotective effects in CNS degenerative diseases and retinal degenerative diseases, including Parkinson's disease (PD) [105], PVR [24], and DR [26]. The following content summarizes the neuroprotective effects of SP in these diseases.

5.1 The protective effect of SP in PD

PD is a slowly progressing movement disorder characterized by tremors, stiffness, and akinesia [106]. This clinical manifestation is primarily due to significant degeneration of dopaminergic neurons in the SN, leading to a 50–70% reduction in tyrosine hydroxylase activity [107]. In addition, studies have shown a decreased dopamine levels in the neostriatum, nucleus accumbens, and frontal cortex of PD patients [108, 109]. Although L-DOPA therapy is a cornerstone of PD patients, a large number of patients either do not maintain a satisfactory response or experience adverse effects [110]. Recent research suggests that neuroprotective therapies, which aim to preserve the integrity and function of vulnerable neurons, might offer significant advantages [111].

Neurons containing SP exhibit close anatomical interactions with the nigrostriatal and midbrain limbic dopaminergic systems [112, 113]. It has also been reported that a dopamine-dependent decrease in SP-like IR levels occurs in postmortem parkinsonian brains, including SN, striatum, and pontine nucleus [114, 115]. Krasnova et al. investigated the effects of intracerebroventricularly administered of SP on dopamine levels and its metabolites in the brain of rats with 6-hydroxydopamine damaged [105]. They found that a higher dose (3.5 nmol/kg) of SP treatment increased the concentration of dopamine, 3,4-dihydroxyphenylacetic acid, and homovanillic acid in the striatum, nucleus accumbens, and frontal cortex, compared to the saline-treated group [105]. These data suggest that SP analogs could potentially have applications in the PD treatment. The mechanism by which SP stimulates dopaminergic neurons is still under investigation. Notably, in PD patients, α-Syn aggregation—a hallmark of the disease, is often co-localized with SP [116]. This observation raises the hypothesis that exogenous SP administration might improve PD symptoms by modulating the abnormal aggregation of α-Syn. Further research is needed to explore this potential neuroprotective effect of SP more comprehensively.

5.2 The protective effect of SP in Alzheimer's disease (AD)

AD is a chronic neurodegenerative disease and is also considered an irreversible neurological disorder [117]. Clinically, AD is characterized by progressive impairment of memory and cognition, accompanied by significant neuronal loss [118]. The hallmark of AD is abnormal extracellular deposition of neurotoxic amyloid-β (Aβ) peptide, which is produced through the proteolytic processing of amyloid precursor protein (APP) [119, 120]. Actually, studies have reported decreased SP levels in the brain tissue of AD patients [121, 122]. In the 1990s, it was proposed that the neuroprotective effect of SP was significantly associated with AD, with *in vitro* studies indicating that SP could reverse the neurotoxic effects of Aβ on hippocampal cells [123]. More recent research has demonstrated that SP can induce APP cleavage, thereby significantly reducing Aβ production without altering the steady-state level of APP [124]. Additionally, upregulation of voltage-gated potassium channel subunits associated with Aβ-induced currents has been implicated in AD pathogenesis [125]. Severini et al. clarified that the protective effect of SP is related to its modulation on Kv channel currents. They showed that SP can reduce Aβ-induced Kv upregulation and restores K^+ current intensity by binding to NK-1R [126].

5.3 The protective effect of SP in DR

The retina, a highly metabolically active tissue, is essential for visual signal transmission [127, 128]. DR is a leading cause of vision loss and blindness, representing a severe complication of diabetes [129]. DR is now understood not only as a microvascular complication of diabetes but also as a neurodegenerative disease [130]. Research has observed that SP expression levels are significantly reduced in diabetic conditions, including in streptozotocin-induced diabetic rat retinas [131] and in the serum of type 1 diabetes patients, particularly those with diabetic neuropathy [132]. These findings suggest a potential involvement of SP in diabetes pathology. Indeed, SP administration has been shown to improve NMDA-induced RGC death and VEGF-induced endothelial cell leakage in the retina, restoring retinal health and inhibiting DR progression [26, 27, 133]. Previous studies indicated that SP levels in the retinas of diabetic rats were significantly reduced, correlating with increased apoptosis of retinal cells and caspase-3 activity. Recovery of endogenous SP levels was associated with reduced RGC apoptosis and caspase-3 activity in diabetic animals [134]. Therefore,

SP likely improves NMDA-induced RGC death by significantly inhibiting caspase-3 activity and cell apoptosis through elevated endogenous SP levels. Furthermore, SP treatment increases the expression of ZO-1 protein and decreases the expression of phosphorylated MAPK (p38 and p44/42) [27, 134], which is known to regulate tight junction function and cellular permeability [135]. This may be a key factor in restoring retinal neurovascular health through SP. Additionally, the barrier function of the RPE is compromised under chronic high glucose (HG) conditions, leading to neovascularization and accelerated DR progression, ultimately resulting in vision loss [136]. Given SP's potential to target the RPE, Lee, Dahyeon, and Hyun Sook Hong investigated whether SP could protect the RPE from HG-induced pathological conditions *in vitro*. They found that SP treatment blocked reductions in cell viability and proliferation, increased tight junction protein expression, and enhanced the antioxidant activity of the RPE, potentially through Akt signaling pathway activation [137]. Moreover, SP treatment decreased the expression of intracellular adhesion molecule-1 (ICAM-1), monocyte chemotactic protein-1 (MCP-1), and VEGF, suggesting its potential application in suppressing inflammation and neovascularization in the RPE [137]. Collectively, these results indicate that SP may be a promising candidate for preventing DR progression, and further studies should evaluate its efficacy in non-clinical animal models.

5.4 The protective effect of SP in PVR

PVR is a leading common cause of repair failure in rhegmatogenous retinal detachment (RRD). It involves the formation of contractile membranes on the detached retinal surface, leading to retinal degeneration and ultimately vision loss [138–140]. Despite studies indicating elevated SP levels in the intraocular fluid of PVR patients [141], SP treatment has been shown to suppress early inflammatory responses, inhibit cell death, and delay retinal degeneration [24]. TNF-α, a prominent inflammatory cytokine, plays a pathogenic role in PVR by affecting RPE cells and inducing morphological changes into fibroblasts [142]. Yoo et al. revealed that SP treatment reduces TNF-α levels, thereby mitigating PVR damage [24], which is consistent with previous reports. Furthermore, SP treatment increases IL-10 [24], coincidence with Carrington et al.'s results showing that IL-10 can inhibit RPE-mediated retinal contraction [143]. These findings suggest that SP exerts its protective effects by exerting anti-inflammatory effects.

5.5 The protective effect of SP in retinal ischemia

SP also shows protective effects in the retinal ischemia [144]. D'Alessandro et al. used mouse model of retinal ischemia to investigate the anti-ischemic potential of SP. They found that SP treatment reduced ischemia-induced cell death, VEGF overexpression, and glutamate release *via* metabolomics analyses [144]. Increased caspase-3 mRNA expression has been previously reported in ischemic retinas [145, 146], but SP treatment was shown to lower caspase-3 mRNA levels, explaining its ability to reduce retinal cell death [144]. Additionally, ischemic state not only leads to cell death, but also induces vascular responses [147]. D'Alessandro et al. observed that SP treatment attenuates the increase in VEGF mRNA levels induced by ischemia [144]. Moreover, as the upstream of caspase-3 [148], SP reduces glutamate excitotoxicity by decreasing glutamate release [144]. These results confirm that SP exerts vital neuroprotective effect in the ischemic retina. Beyond the retina, SP also demonstrates cardioprotective effects following ischemia-reperfusion, attributed to its potent coronary vasodilation effects and its activation of AKT pathways in myocardial cells, mediated through NK-1R [149, 150]. Additionally, SP's immunomodulatory properties can improve renal ischemia-reperfusion injury and prevent kidney disease progression [151].

5.6 The protective effect of SP in age-related macular degeneration (AMD)

The RPE is a monolayer of cells situated between the choroid and the outer segments of photoreceptor cells. Its primary functions include providing nutrients to photoreceptor cells, phagocytosing photoreceptor outer segments, and facilitating the transfer of waste products from retina to the choroidal vascular system [152]. The normal structure and function of RPE are crucial for maintaining retinal health [153]. However, as aging, ROS accumulates in the choroid, RPE, and retina. These ROS can damage the RPE, leading to chronic inflammation, structural damage, and functional impairment of the RPE, which contributes to the development of AMD [154–156]. AMD, a leading cause of vision loss, becomes increasingly prevalent with age [157]. Despite its complex pathogenesis, there is currently no ideal treatment for AMD. Recent studies have highlighted the anti-inflammatory effects of SP, including its ability to ameliorate collagen II-induced arthritis in mice and convert M1 macrophages to the anti-inflammatory M2 phenotype [158, 159]. Given the role of inflammation in AMD progression, Hong et al. investigated the potential of SP to protect against retinal degeneration. They used an argon laser to induce RPE injury and evaluated SP's protective effects by assessing retinal integrity, neovascularization, and serum cytokine levels [160]. SP treatment was found to reduce TNF-α levels and increase IL-10 levels in the serum, suggesting that SP inhibits early-stage inflammation [160]. Additionally, SP was shown to block apoptosis caused by laser-induced retinal injury and reduce abnormal retinal vascularization [160]. Furthermore, given that cell survival requires activation of Akt signaling under oxidative stress [161, 162], SP usually relies on the mediation of NK-1R to exert its function. Baek et al. explored the antioxidant effects of SP on RPE cells damaged by H_2O_2. Their *in vitro* results indicated that SP suppresses cell viability reduction, enhances cell proliferation, and decreases cell apoptosis [163]. They also found that SP activates Akt/GSK-3β signaling through NK-1R, thereby protecting RPE cells from oxidative stress-induced cell death [163]. Their findings suggest that SP could be a promising therapeutic option for AMD and other inflammatory/oxidative stress-related ocular diseases.

5.7 Controversies surrounding the protective role of SP

While many studies support the potential of SP as a therapeutic agent for retinal diseases, there are conflicting data. Some research indicates that SP can induce endothelial cells to produce nitric oxide or interact with granulocytes and mast cells to regulate angiogenesis, and that blocking the VEGF signaling pathway does not negate SP's proangiogenic effects [164–166]. Additionally, elevated SP levels have been observed in patients with type 2 diabetes, particularly those with proliferative diabetic retinopathy (PDR) [167]. Variations in SP expression levels and effects may be attributed to differences in disease types, stages, and experimental methodologies. Consequently, further research is needed to validate the neuroprotective effects of SP and assess its effectiveness and safety for potential use in treating various retinal diseases.

6. The role of SP in the CNS diseases

6.1 SP exerts an immunomodulatory role in the CNS

SP plays an important role in various pathophysiological processes within the human nervous system, including pain transmission, neurodegenerative diseases, inflammatory processes, and the enhancement of the blood-brain barrier permeability. These effects are largely mediated through its immunomodulation to function.

In the CNS, SP exerts an immunomodulatory role by shifting it toward Th17 immunity and by regulating the Th1/Th2 balance based on the nature of the antigen. In addition to its effects on Th1 and Th2 cells, SP also influences the inflammatory response to favor Th17 immunity [168].

6.2 SP is involved in pain transmission

SP excessive release or altered processing may contribute to neuropathic pain conditions where chronic pain arises from nerve damage or dysfunction [169]. In studies involving mice with a disrupted NK-1R gene, it was observed that these mice, despite being healthy and hypertrophied and capable of normal reproduction, lacked the characteristic amplification and intensity of nociceptive reflexes. This suggests that SP's peripheral release contributes to neurogenic inflammatory responses [170]. When capsaicin, a neurotoxin that eliminates over 90% of sensory afferent nerve fibers, was applied to the ears of NK-1R knockout mice, a 74% reduction in inflammation was observed compared to the control group [170]. Additionally, following carrageenan injection into the hind paw, the inflammatory response was reduced by 62% in the NK-1R knockout mice compared to controls. SP expression in sensory subsets of spinal cord neurons increased after inflammatory injury, suggesting that elevated SP levels may lead to central sensitization and hyperalgesia associated with inflammation [171, 172]. Further studies exploring the relationship between analgesia and SP involved low-dose morphine administration. This resulted in an increased hot plate threshold in both $NK1^{+/+}$ and $NK1^{-/-}$ animals, but in $NK1^{-/-}$ mice, low-dose morphine significantly reduced the increase in the tail flick threshold, suggesting that SP partially mediates opioid-induced modulation of spinal cord reflexes [173–176]. Thus, while SP may not directly mediate acute pain or analgesia, it plays a crucial role in the adaptive pain response, highlighting its unexpected importance in inflammation and pain management [169].

6.3 SP plays an important role in neurodegenerative diseases

In a study examining the role of SP in patients with AD, it was found that SP can stimulate non-amyloid processing of APP, thereby reducing the production of toxic Aβ peptides in the brain. Both *in vitro* and *in vivo* models have suggested that SP's neuroprotective effect on Aβ might be related to its ability to regulate Kv channel currents [126]. In the cerebral cortex of healthy individuals, there are neurons, deep in the cortex, and rich in NADPH phosphatase that produce SP and its precursor mRNA. These neurons are surprisingly depleted in AD, in contrast to other local circuit neurons, suggesting that they may be early targets for degenerative processes. In the human basal ganglia, SP and its corresponding mRNA are localized to certain neurons within the globus pallidus. In patients with PD, SP and mRNA are enriched in D1 dopamine receptors and abnormal proteins, and a subset of spinous striated local circuit neurons also contains SP [177]. In Huntington's disease, SP levels are depleted in striatum neurons. Staining data reveal a gradual depletion of SP in neurons of globus pallidus and SN, accompanied by stripe atrophy. While these neurons exhibit resistance to degeneration in Huntington's disease, they are more susceptible to degeneration in AD. The localization of the SP receptor in the globus pallidus or SN in humans remains unclear. These findings underscore the close association between neurodegenerative diseases [178].

6.4 SP is involved in inflammatory processes

SP is implicated in neuroinflammatory diseases such as multiple sclerosis (MS) [179], AD [126], and PD [177]. MS is an autoimmune disease characterized by inflammatory responses and demyelination within the CNS, which progress over time. The clinical manifestations involve an immune response to myelin components triggered by environmental factors or nonspecific viral infections. This response ultimately leads to the release of SP and the expression of its receptor. The transition from the inflammatory phase to demyelination and glial hyperplasia can exacerbate MS. Additionally, interaction between SP receptors on neurons may influence disease progression in different individuals [179]. Consequently, SP and its receptors represent potential therapeutic targets for controlling disease progression, especially with the availability of non-toxic SP antagonists [180].

6.5 SP enhances the permeability of the blood-brain barrier

SP enhances blood-brain barrier (BBB) permeability by disrupting tight junction proteins [181], thereby contributing to MS [179] and edema following traumatic brain injury (TBI) [182], spinal cord injury (SCI), and stroke [183].

In MS, SP interacts with astrocytes and oligodendrocytes, increasing BBB permeability and allowing the influx of immune mediators and activated T cells [184, 185]. This influx leads to further release of cytokines and SP, which then acts on major cellular components of the MS plaque—lymphocytes, macrophages, and glial cells—through specific receptors, driving a proliferative and pro-inflammatory response [179].

Following TBI, SP expression increases and binds to NK-1Rs, inducing neuroinflammation and further increasing BBB permeability, which raises intracranial pressure and results in poor clinical outcomes. NK-1R antagonists have been shown to reduce cerebral edema and intracranial pressure in animal models of TBI [182].

Clinical studies reveal elevated SP levels in cerebrospinal fluid (CSF) in patients with SCI [186]. SP levels are significantly increased at 5 mm from the injury site at 1 and 2 hours post-thoracic injury, with further increases observed in the brain at 5 hours after injury [187]. Regulation of SP following spinal cord trauma appears to occur throughout the CNS, as demonstrated in animal experiments. For instance, SP levels increased significantly after T12 spinal cord transection in female cats [188]. Conversely, rodent models of SCI showed a decrease in SP at the injury site [189]. Additionally, NK-1R expression was significantly elevated 1 week post-injury in rat SCI models [190]. These changes suggest that SP plays a role in the pathogenesis of SCI and its complications.

In stroke patients, SP levels are associated with significant BBB disruption, as evidenced by increased extravasation of Evans blue dye into brain parenchyma 24 hours post-stroke [191]. Deep cerebral edema is also linked to increased BBB permeability, indicating vascular involvement [192]. Given the documented increases in SP in stroke studies, researchers have explored NK-1R antagonists as a means to mitigate BBB dysfunction and vasogenic edema in ischemic stroke [192]. Yu and colleagues reported reduced infarct size and improved neurological outcomes 24 hours post-stroke with the administration of the NK-1R antagonist SR-14033 [193]. Robert Vink's study further supports the efficacy of NK-1R antagonists in experimental ischemic stroke, demonstrating that intravenous NK-1R antagonist therapy 4 hours after stroke can reduce cerebral edema [192]. When combined with tissue plasminogen activator (tPA) therapy, NK-1R antagonists performed comparably or better in functional outcome tests than either NK-1R antagonists or tPA alone [194].

The dense distribution of perivascular sensory nerve fibers in the cerebrovascular system allows for rapid neurogenic inflammation following cerebrovascular injury. Elevated perivascular SP, in conjunction with other neuropeptides, contributes to increased vascular permeability, vasodilation, and edema formation. Inhibiting post-traumatic neurogenic inflammation through neuropeptide release suppression or NK-1R antagonism can prevent BBB disruption and edema formation, making NK-1R a promising therapeutic target for these conditions [195].

6.6 SP plays a crucial role in retina diseases

SP is increasingly recognized for its significant role in various retinal diseases. Here is an overview of how SP is implicated in these conditions:

In PVR, SP notably delays retinal degeneration. It achieves this by inhibiting the early inflammatory response—specifically, by decreasing TNF-α levels and increasing IL-10, thereby reducing cell death and the emergence of fibroblasts. Furthermore, SP mitigates TNF-α-induced epithelial-to-mesenchymal transition (EMT) in RPE cells and directly prevents fibrotic changes in these cells [196]. Previous research has demonstrated that dispase injections can damage blood vessels by destroying the inner limiting membrane and penetrating the retina. This damage triggers inflammation not only in the vitreous and retina but also in the anterior chamber, leading to fibrosis and retinal detachment [197, 198]. When the retina detaches, the RPE layer becomes dysfunctional, resulting in reduced retinal cell viability and degeneration [199–201]. In experiments designed to induce PVR-like retinal disease, dispase is injected intravitreally while SP is administered systemically [24]. Histological analysis conducted 1 week after dispase injection revealed that severe structural damage was rarely observed in both the control and SP-treated groups, with the retinal layers largely intact [24]. Analysis of cell density in the inner nuclear layer (INL) and outer nuclear layer (ONL) indicated that while dispase injection slightly reduced cell viability in these layers, SP treatment effectively countered this effect. $CD31^+$ vasculature, indicative of new blood vessel formation, was present in the control group but was slightly reduced in the SP-treated group [24]. Three weeks post-dispase injection, the control group exhibited significant disruption of retinal structures and blurred boundaries between the INL and ONL, whereas SP treatment notably mitigated retinal damage. Quantitative analysis confirmed that SP treatment significantly prevented dispase-induced cell loss in both the ONL and INL [138].

Retinal folding is an early sign of PVR that progresses to form a fibrous membrane, leading to structural changes in retinal cells [198]. The retina in the control group exhibited complex folds and rosette-like cellular invaginations, while the SP-treated group showed a more intact INL and ONL with fewer folds. These findings suggest that SP can inhibit the progression of dispase-induced retinal damage by preventing retinal folding and preserving cell viability [24].

Clinical studies have revealed that patients undergoing secondary cataract surgery on their second eye often experience more pain compared to their first eye surgery. This increased pain is partly attributed to elevated MCP-1 levels in the aqueous humor. Additionally, experiments have shown that SP is involved in the sympathetic nerve inflammatory response of the contralateral eye in patients with type II diabetes [202, 203]. After cataract surgery in the first eye, increased levels of SP and MCP-1 were detected in the contralateral eyelid layer, indicating that both SP and MCP-1 contribute to the sympathetic inflammatory response [204, 205]. This also suggests that diabetic patients are more susceptible to non-infectious inflammation following cataract surgery and experience more pain during phacoemulsification of the second eye [25].

In DR, chronic inflammation plays a critical role in disease progression. Research on SP's effects on glucose metabolism, lipid metabolism, systemic inflammation, and retinopathy involved using Otsuka Long-Evans Tokushima Fatty (OLETF) rats, which exhibit chronic inflammation, obesity, and impaired bone marrow stem cell function [206]. These rats display typical type 2 diabetes mellitus (T2DM) symptoms, such as obesity, chronic inflammation, and poor glycemic control [207]. SP treatment in these rats inhibited weight gain, reduced levels of circulating free fatty acids, cholesterol, and triglycerides, and improved the obesity environment. SP also mitigated the inflammatory response and rejuvenated bone marrow stem cells [208]. Additionally, SP's metabolic and immune effects address hyperglycemia and insulin resistance. Histological findings revealed that SP treatment alleviated dysfunction in insulin resistance target tissues. Although OLETF rats exhibited retinal damage at 27 weeks, worsening by 31 weeks [209], SP treatment restored the damaged retina to a structure similar to that of non-diabetic rats [210]. Thus, systemic SP application helps inhibit the progression of type 2 diabetes and DR, influencing inflammatory pathways and contributing to vascular and neuronal changes observed in DR [26].

In retinal diseases such as retinal vein occlusion and PDR, the blood-retinal barrier (BRB) is compromised due to factors such as hypoxia and increased VEGF, leading to retinal edema and neovascularization [211]. Dysregulation of neurovascular integrity in the retina is a key factor in RGC death and vision loss [212]. Experiments involving NMDA-induced RGC excitotoxic apoptosis and VEGF-induced retinal vascular leakage in *ex vivo* and mouse models explored whether SP could inhibit NMDA and provide protective effects on RGCs. Following NMDA administration, a reduction in TUNEL+ cells was observed, while Brn-3a + cell numbers remained unchanged, indicating SP's inhibitory effect on RGC apoptosis [213]. Additionally, SP was found to maintain endothelial tight junctions and reduce VEGF-induced permeability, suggesting a protective role against NMDA-induced apoptosis and VEGF-induced endothelial barrier disruption in RGCs [27].

SP also promotes the survival of retinal neurons by inhibiting inflammation and neoangiogenesis [214]. This is particularly relevant in AMD [156, 215], where retinal degeneration is driven by neoangiogenesis and persistent inflammation of the RPE and choroid [216]. Inhibition of these processes is crucial for protecting the retina from degeneration. One week after argon laser damage to the retina in mice, the SP treatment group exhibited lower TNF-α and IL-10 serum concentrations and maintained more intact retinal structures compared to the vehicle treatment group. Mice that received SP for 4 weeks showed normal retinal structures and sparse neoangiogenesis, whereas the control group experienced severe retinal disruption and dense neoangiogenesis. SP demonstrated comparable efficacy to MSCs transplanted into the vitreous following retinal injury [217]. These findings underscore the potential of endogenous neuropeptide SP as a treatment to prevent retinal damage and diseases such as AMD [160].

Funding

This work was supported in part by grants from the National Key Research and Development Program of China (2022YFA1105503), State Key Laboratory of Neuroscience (SKLN-202103), Zhejiang Natural Science Foundation of China (LY21H120004), The High-Level Innovation Team Program of Wenzhou (88923002), Zhejiang Provincial Health Commission Foundation of China (2021KY809).

Author details

Fenglan Wang[1,2], Zhongqun Chen[1,2], Guiyu Guan[1,2] and Jun Zhang[1,2]*

1 The State Key Laboratory of Ophthalmology, Optometry and Visual Science, Wenzhou Medical University, Wenzhou, China

2 Laboratory of Retinal Physiology and Disease, Eye Hospital and School of Ophthalmology and Optometry, Wenzhou Medical University, Wenzhou, China

*Address all correspondence to: zj9999@eye.ac.cn

References

[1] Us VE, Gaddum JH. An unidentified depressor substance in certain tissue extracts. The Journal of Physiology. 1931;**72**(1):74-87

[2] Chang MM, Leeman SE. Isolation of a sialogogic peptide from bovine hypothalamic tissue and its characterization as substance P. The Journal of Biological Chemistry. 1970;**245**(18):4784-4790

[3] Severini C, Improta G, Falconieri-Erspamer G, et al. The tachykinin peptide family. Pharmacological Reviews. 2002;**54**(2):285-322

[4] Krause JE, Chirgwin JM, Carter MS, et al. Three rat preprotachykinin mRNAs encode the neuropeptides substance P and neurokinin a. Proceedings of the National Academy of Sciences of the United States of America. 1987;**84**(3):881-885

[5] Nawa H, Hirose T, Takashima H, et al. Nucleotide sequences of cloned cDNAs for two types of bovine brain substance P precursor. Nature. 1983;**306**(5938):32-36

[6] Hökfelt T, Johansson O, Ljungdahl A, et al. Peptidergic neurones. Nature. 1980;**284**(5756):515-521

[7] Michel JP, Sakamoto N, Bouvier R, et al. Substance P-immunoreactive astrocytes related to deep white matter and striatal blood vessels in human brain. Brain Research. 1986;**377**(2):383-387

[8] Lai JP, Zhan GX, Campbell DE, et al. Detection of substance P and its receptor in human fetal microglia. Neuroscience. 2000;**101**(4):1137-1144

[9] Watanabe M, Nakayasu K, Iwatsu M, et al. Endogenous substance P in corneal epithelial cells and keratocytes. Japanese Journal of Ophthalmology. 2002;**46**(6):616-620

[10] Bowden JJ, Baluk P, Lefevre PM, et al. Substance P (NK1) receptor immunoreactivity on endothelial cells of the rat tracheal mucosa. The American Journal of Physiology. 1996;**270**(3 Pt. 1):L404-L414

[11] Chang MM, Leeman SE, Niall HD. Amino-acid sequence of substance P. Nature: New Biology. 1971;**232**(29):86-87

[12] Mashaghi A, Marmalidou A, Tehrani M, et al. Neuropeptide substance P and the immune response. Cellular and Molecular Life Sciences. 2016;**73**(22):4249-4264

[13] Mcgregor GP, Bloom SR. Radioimmunoassay of substance P and its stability in tissue. Life Sciences. 1983;**32**(6):655-662

[14] XanthosDN, SandkühlerJ. Neurogenic neuroinflammation: Inflammatory CNS reactions in response to neuronal activity. Nature Reviews. Neuroscience. 2014;**15**(1):43-53

[15] Pavlova MN, Kaz'min AI, Abal'masova EA, et al. Pathomorphological characteristics of the intervertebral disks in scoliosis of varying etiology. Ortopediia Travmatologiia i Protezirovanie. 1976;**10**:1-7

[16] O'connor TM, O'connell J, O'brien DI, et al. The role of substance P in inflammatory disease. Journal of Cellular Physiology. 2004;**201**(2):167-180

[17] Zhu J, Qu C, Lu X, et al. Activation of microglia by histamine and substance

P. Cellular Physiology and Biochemistry. 2014;**34**(3):768-780

[18] Zhou Z, Barrett RP, Mcclellan SA, et al. Substance P delays apoptosis, enhancing keratitis after *Pseudomonas aeruginosa* infection. Investigative Ophthalmology & Visual Science. 2008;**49**(10):4458-4467

[19] Ziche M, Morbidelli L, Pacini M, et al. Substance P stimulates neovascularization in vivo and proliferation of cultured endothelial cells. Microvascular Research. 1990;**40**(2):264-278

[20] Zalutsky RA, Miller RF. The physiology of substance P in the rabbit retina. The Journal of Neuroscience. 1990;**10**(2):394-402

[21] Casini G, Dal Monte M, Fornai F, et al. Neurokinin 1 receptor expression and substance P physiological actions are developmentally regulated in the rabbit retina. Neuroscience. 2004;**124**(1):147-160

[22] Almeida TA, Rojo J, Nieto PM, et al. Tachykinins and tachykinin receptors: Structure and activity relationships. Current Medicinal Chemistry. 2004;**11**(15):2045-2081

[23] Kondoh A, Houtani T, Ueyama T, et al. In situ hybridization analysis of substance P receptor in the rat retina. Experimental Brain Research. 1996;**112**(2):181-186

[24] Yoo K, Son BK, Kim S, et al. Substance P prevents development of proliferative vitreoretinopathy in mice by modulating TNF-α. Molecular Vision. 2017;**23**:933-943

[25] Gong X, Ren Y, Fang X, et al. Substance P induces sympathetic immune response in the contralateral eye after the first eye cataract surgery in type 2 diabetic patients. BMC Ophthalmology. 2020;**20**(1):339

[26] Baek SM, Kim K, Kim S, et al. SP prevents T2DM complications by immunomodulation. Scientific Reports. 2020;**10**(1):16753

[27] Ou K, Mertsch S, Theodoropoulou S, et al. Restoring retinal neurovascular health via substance P. Experimental Cell Research. 2019;**380**(2):115-123

[28] Pickel VM, Reis DJ, Leeman SE. Ultrastructural localization of substance P in neurons of rat spinal cord. Brain Research. 1977;**122**(3):534-540

[29] Lai JP, Douglas SD, Ho WZ. Human lymphocytes express substance P and its receptor. Journal of Neuroimmunology. 1998;**86**(1):80-86

[30] Milner P, Bodin P, Guiducci S, et al. Regulation of substance P mRNA expression in human dermal microvascular endothelial cells. Clinical and Experimental Rheumatology. 2004;**22**(3 Suppl. 33):S24-S27

[31] Marriott I, Bost KL. IL-4 and IFN-gamma up-regulate substance P receptor expression in murine peritoneal macrophages. Journal of Immunology. 2000;**165**(1):182-191

[32] Lambrecht BN, Germonpré PR, Everaert EG, et al. Endogenously produced substance P contributes to lymphocyte proliferation induced by dendritic cells and direct TCR ligation. European Journal of Immunology. 1999;**29**(12):3815-3825

[33] Weinstock JV, Blum A, Walder J, et al. Eosinophils from granulomas in murine schistosomiasis mansoni produce substance P. Journal of Immunology. 1988;**141**(3):961-966

[34] Cho KJ, Trzaska KA, Greco SJ, et al. Neurons derived from human mesenchymal stem cells show synaptic transmission and can be induced to produce the neurotransmitter substance P by interleukin-1 alpha. Stem Cells. 2005;**23**(3):383-391

[35] Monastyrskaya K, Hostettler A, Buergi S, et al. The NK1 receptor localizes to the plasma membrane microdomains, and its activation is dependent on lipid raft integrity. The Journal of Biological Chemistry. 2005;**280**(8):7135-7146

[36] Fong TM, Anderson SA, Yu H, et al. Differential activation of intracellular effector by two isoforms of human neurokinin-1 receptor. Molecular Pharmacology. 1992;**41**(1):24-30

[37] Todd AJ, Mcgill MM, Shehab SA. Neurokinin 1 receptor expression by neurons in laminae I, III and IV of the rat spinal dorsal horn that project to the brainstem. The European Journal of Neuroscience. 2000;**12**(2):689-700

[38] Chauhan VS, Sterka DG Jr, DL G, et al. Neurogenic exacerbation of microglial and astrocyte responses to Neisseria meningitidis and *Borrelia burgdorferi*. Journal of Immunology. 2008;**180**(12):8241-8249

[39] Böckmann S, Substance P. (NK(1)) receptor expression by human colonic epithelial cell line Caco-2. Peptides. 2002;**23**(10):1783-1791

[40] Greeno EW, Mantyh P, Vercellotti GM, et al. Functional neurokinin 1 receptors for substance P are expressed by human vascular endothelium. The Journal of Experimental Medicine. 1993;**177**(5):1269-1276

[41] Maghni K, Michoud MC, Alles M, et al. Airway smooth muscle cells express functional neurokinin-1 receptors and the nerve-derived preprotachykinin-A gene: Regulation by passive sensitization. American Journal of Respiratory Cell and Molecular Biology. 2003;**28**(1):103-110

[42] Liu JY, Hu JH, Zhu QG, et al. Substance P receptor expression in human skin keratinocytes and fibroblasts. The British Journal of Dermatology. 2006;**155**(4):657-662

[43] Feistritzer C, Clausen J, Sturn DH, et al. Natural killer cell functions mediated by the neuropeptide substance P. Regulatory Peptides. 2003;**116**(1-3):119-126

[44] Marriott I, Bost KL. Expression of authentic substance P receptors in murine and human dendritic cells. Journal of Neuroimmunology. 2001;**114**(1-2):131-141

[45] Germonpre PR, Bullock GR, Lambrecht BN, et al. Presence of substance P and neurokinin 1 receptors in human sputum macrophages and U-937 cells. The European Respiratory Journal. 1999;**14**(4):776-782

[46] Van Der Kleij HP, Ma D, Redegeld FA, et al. Functional expression of neurokinin 1 receptors on mast cells induced by IL-4 and stem cell factor. Journal of Immunology. 2003;**171**(4):2074-2079

[47] Cuello AC, Kanazawa I. The distribution of substance P immunoreactive fibers in the rat central nervous system. The Journal of Comparative Neurology. 1978;**178**(1):129-156

[48] Lembeck F, Holzer P. Substance P as neurogenic mediator of antidromic vasodilation and neurogenic plasma extravasation. Naunyn-Schmiedeberg's Archives of Pharmacology. 1979;**310**(2):175-183

[49] Paasonen MK, Vogt M. The effect of drugs on the amounts of substance P and 5-hydroxytryptamine in mammalian brain. The Journal of Physiology. 1956;**131**(3):617-626

[50] Ribeiro-Da-Silva A, Hökfelt T. Neuroanatomical localisation of substance P in the CNS and sensory neurons. Neuropeptides. 2000;**34**(5):256-271

[51] Douglas SD, Leeman SE. Neurokinin-1 receptor: Functional significance in the immune system in reference to selected infections and inflammation. Annals of the New York Academy of Sciences. 2011;**1217**:83-95

[52] Ebner K, Singewald N. The role of substance P in stress and anxiety responses. Amino Acids. 2006;**31**(3):251-272

[53] Fukuda M, Kuwayama Y, Shiosaka S, et al. Demonstration of a substance P-like immunoreactivity in retinal cells of the rat. Neuroscience Letters. 1981;**23**(3):239-242

[54] Wang F, Zhong W, Yang Q, et al. Distribution and synaptic organization of substance P-like immunoreactive neurons in the mouse retina. Brain Structure & Function. 2023;**228**(7):1703-1724

[55] Yazulla S, Studholme KM, Zucker CL. Synaptic organization of substance P-like immunoreactive amacrine cells in goldfish retina. The Journal of Comparative Neurology. 1985;**231**(2):232-238

[56] Li HB, So KF, Cheuk W. Substance P-immunoreactive neurons in hamster retinas. Visual Neuroscience. 1999;**16**(3):475-481

[57] Brecha N, Johnson D, Bolz J, et al. Substance P-immunoreactive retinal ganglion cells and their central axon terminals in the rabbit. Nature. 1987;**327**(6118):155-158

[58] Pourcho RG, Goebel DJ. Substance P-like immunoreactive amacrine cells in the cat retina. The Journal of Comparative Neurology. 1988;**275**(4):542-552

[59] Watt CB, Florack VJ. Colocalization of glycine in substance P-amacrine cells of the larval tiger salamander retina. Visual Neuroscience. 1993;**10**(5):899-906

[60] Lee MY, Chun MH, Han SH, et al. Light- and electron-microscopic study of substance P-immunoreactive neurons in the Guinea pig retina. Cell and Tissue Research. 1995;**281**(2):261-271

[61] Brecha N, Hendrickson A, Florén I, et al. Localization of substance P-like immunoreactivity within the monkey retina. Investigative Ophthalmology & Visual Science. 1982;**23**(2):147-153

[62] Cuenca N, De Juan J, Kolb H. Substance P-immunoreactive neurons in the human retina. The Journal of Comparative Neurology. 1995;**356**(4):491-504

[63] Dick E, Miller RF. Peptides influence retinal ganglion cells. Neuroscience Letters. 1981;**26**(2):131-135

[64] Glickman RD, Adolph AR. Acetylcholine and substance P: Action via distinct receptors on carp retinal ganglion cells. Investigative Ophthalmology & Visual Science. 1982;**22**(6):804-808

[65] Cuenca N, Kolb H. Morphology and distribution of neurons immunoreactive for substance P in the turtle retina. The Journal of Comparative Neurology. 1989;**290**(3):391-411

[66] Pourcho RG. Dopaminergic amacrine cells in the cat retina. Brain Research. 1982;**252**(1):101-109

[67] Voigt T, Wässle H. Dopaminergic innervation of A II amacrine cells in mammalian retina. The Journal of Neuroscience. 1987;7(12):4115-4128

[68] Dacey RG Jr, Bassett JE, Takayasu M. Vasomotor responses of rat intracerebral arterioles to vasoactive intestinal peptide, substance P, neuropeptide Y, and bradykinin. Journal of Cerebral Blood Flow and Metabolism. 1988;**8**(2):254-261

[69] Dacey DM. The dopaminergic amacrine cell. The Journal of Comparative Neurology. 1990;**301**(3):461-489

[70] Kolb H, Cuenca N, Wang HH, et al. The synaptic organization of the dopaminergic amacrine cell in the cat retina. Journal of Neurocytology. 1990;**19**(3):343-366

[71] Kolb H, Cuenca N, Dekorver L. Postembedding immunocytochemistry for GABA and glycine reveals the synaptic relationships of the dopaminergic amacrine cell of the cat retina. The Journal of Comparative Neurology. 1991;**310**(2):267-284

[72] Cuenca N, Kolb H. Circuitry and role of substance P-immunoreactive neurons in the primate retina. The Journal of Comparative Neurology. 1998;**393**(4):439-456

[73] Denis P, Fardin V, Nordmann JP, et al. Localization and characterization of substance P binding sites in rat and rabbit eyes. Investigative Ophthalmology & Visual Science. 1991;**32**(6):1894-1902

[74] Caberlotto L, Hurd YL, Murdock P, et al. Neurokinin 1 receptor and relative abundance of the short and long isoforms in the human brain. The European Journal of Neuroscience. 2003;**17**(9):1736-1746

[75] Andoh T, Nagasawa T, Kuraishi Y. Expression of tachykinin NK1 receptor mRNA in dorsal root ganglia of the mouse. Brain Research. Molecular Brain Research. 1996;**35**(1-2):329-332

[76] Hietala J, Nyman MJ, Eskola O, et al. Visualization and quantification of neurokinin-1 (NK1) receptors in the human brain. Molecular Imaging and Biology. 2005;**7**(4):262-272

[77] Garcia-Recio S, Gascón P. Biological and pharmacological aspects of the NK1-receptor. BioMed Research International. 2015;**2015**:495704

[78] Liu H, Brown JL, Jasmin L, et al. Synaptic relationship between substance P and the substance P receptor: Light and electron microscopic characterization of the mismatch between neuropeptides and their receptors. Proceedings of the National Academy of Sciences of the United States of America. 1994;**91**(3):1009-1013

[79] Casini G, Rickman DW, Sternini C, et al. Neurokinin 1 receptor expression in the rat retina. The Journal of Comparative Neurology. 1997;**389**(3):496-507

[80] Oyamada H, Takatsuji K, Senba E, et al. Postnatal development of NK1, NK2, and NK3 neurokinin receptors expression in the rat retina. Brain Research. Developmental Brain Research. 1999;**117**(1):59-70

[81] Casini G, Brecha NC, Bosco L, et al. Developmental expression of neurokinin-1 and neurokinin-3 receptors in the rat retina. The Journal of Comparative Neurology. 2000;**421**(2):275-287

[82] Catalani E, Gangitano C, Bosco L, et al. Expression of the neurokinin 1 receptor in the mouse retina. Neuroscience. 2004;**128**(3):519-530

[83] Casini G, Sabatini A, Catalani E, et al. Expression of the neurokinin 1 receptor in the rabbit retina. Neuroscience. 2002;**115**(4):1309-1321

[84] Bolam JP, Smith Y. The GABA and substance P input to dopaminergic neurones in the substantia nigra of the rat. Brain Research. 1990;**529**(1-2):57-78

[85] Caruso DM, Owczarzak MT, Pourcho RG. Colocalization of substance P and GABA in retinal ganglion cells: A computer-assisted visualization. Visual Neuroscience. 1990;**5**(4):389-394

[86] Caruso DM, Owczarzak MT, Goebel DJ, et al. GABA-immunoreactivity in ganglion cells of the rat retina. Brain Research. 1989;**476**(1):129-134

[87] Pourcho RG, Goebel DJ. Colocalization of substance P and gamma-aminobutyric acid in amacrine cells of the cat retina. Brain Research. 1988;**447**(1):164-168

[88] Nicholas AP, Pieribone VA, Arvidsson U, et al. Serotonin-, substance P- and glutamate/aspartate-like immunoreactivities in medullo-spinal pathways of rat and primate. Neuroscience. 1992;**48**(3):545-559

[89] Hökfelt T, Vincent S, Dalsgaard CJ, et al. Distribution of substance P in brain and periphery and its possible role as a co-transmitter. Ciba Foundation Symposium. 1982;**91**:84-106

[90] Arvidsson U, Cullheim S, Ulfhake B, et al. 5-Hydroxytryptamine, substance P, and thyrotropin-releasing hormone in the adult cat spinal cord segment L7: Immunohistochemical and chemical studies. Synapse. 1990;**6**(3):237-270

[91] Graefe SB, Rahimi N, Mohiuddin SS. Biochemistry, Substance P. In: StatPearls [Internet]. Treasure Island (FL): StatPearls Publishing; 30 Jul 2023

[92] Devane CL. Substance P: A new era, a new role. Pharmacotherapy. 2001;**21**(9):1061-1069

[93] Dasgupta A, Baby N, Krishna K, et al. Substance P induces plasticity and synaptic tagging/capture in rat hippocampal area CA2. Proceedings of the National Academy of Sciences of the United States of America. 2017;**114**(41):E8741-E87e9

[94] Kouznetsova M, Nistri A. Modulation by substance P of synaptic transmission in the mouse hippocampal slice. The European Journal of Neuroscience. 1998;**10**(10):3076-3084

[95] Ogier R, Raggenbass M. Action of tachykinins in the rat hippocampus: Modulation of inhibitory synaptic transmission. The European Journal of Neuroscience. 2003;**17**(12):2639-2647

[96] Chevaleyre V, Siegelbaum SA. Strong CA2 pyramidal neuron synapses define a powerful disynaptic cortico-hippocampal loop. Neuron. 2010;**66**(4):560-572

[97] Bolam JP, Izzo PN. The postsynaptic targets of substance P-immunoreactive terminals in the rat neostriatum with particular reference to identified spiny striatonigral neurons. Experimental Brain Research. 1988;**70**(2):361-377

[98] He ZX, Liu TY, Yin YY, et al. Substance P plays a critical role in synaptic transmission in striatal neurons. Biochemical and Biophysical Research Communications. 2019;**511**(2):369-373

[99] Melani R, Von Itter R, Jing D, et al. Opposing effects of an atypical glycinergic and substance P transmission on interpeduncular nucleus plasticity. Neuropsychopharmacology: Official Publication of the American College of Neuropsychopharmacology. 2019;**44**(10):1828-1836

[100] Yamaguchi K, Nakajima Y, Nakajima S, et al. Modulation of inwardly rectifying channels by substance P in cholinergic neurones from rat brain in culture. The Journal of Physiology. 1990;**426**:499-520

[101] Glickman RD, Adolph AR, Dowling JE. Inner plexiform circuits in the carp retina: Effects of cholinergic agonists, GABA, and substance P on the ganglion cells. Brain Research. 1982;**234**(1):81-99

[102] Ayoub GS, Matthews G. Substance P modulates calcium current in retinal bipolar neurons. Visual Neuroscience. 1992;**8**(6):539-544

[103] Nawy S, Von Gersdorff H. Bipolar cells in the vertebrate retina: From form to function. Introduction. Visual Neuroscience. 2011;**28**(1):1-2

[104] Bley KR, Tsien RW. Inhibition of Ca2+ and K+ channels in sympathetic neurons by neuropeptides and other ganglionic transmitters. Neuron. 1990;**4**(3):379-391

[105] Krasnova IN, Bychkov ER, Lioudyno VI, et al. Intracerebroventricular administration of substance P increases dopamine content in the brain of 6-hydroxydopamine-lesioned rats. Neuroscience. 2000;**95**(1):113-117

[106] Yenilmez F, Fründt O, Hidding U, et al. Cannabis in Parkinson's disease: The Patients' view. Journal of Parkinson's Disease. 2021;**11**(1):309-321

[107] Javoy-Agid F, Agid Y. Is the mesocortical dopaminergic system involved in Parkinson disease? Neurology. 1980;**30**(12):1326-1330

[108] Scatton B, Javoy-Agid F, Rouquier L, et al. Reduction of cortical dopamine, noradrenaline, serotonin and their metabolites in Parkinson's disease. Brain Research. 1983;**275**(2):321-328

[109] Paulson GW, Aotsuka A. Parkinsonian syndromes. Seminars in Neurology. 1993;**13**(4):359-364

[110] Ogawa N. Levodopa and dopamine agonists in the treatment of Parkinson's disease: Advantages and disadvantages. European Neurology. 1994;**34** (Suppl. 3):20-28

[111] Koller WC. Neuroprotective therapy for Parkinson's disease. Experimental Neurology. 1997;**144**(1):24-28

[112] Mendez I, Elisevich K, Flumerfelt B. Substance P synaptic interactions with GABAergic and dopaminergic neurons in rat substantia nigra: An ultrastructural double-labeling immunocytochemical study. Brain Research Bulletin. 1992;**28**(4):557-563

[113] Pickel VM, Joh TH, Chan J. Substance P in the rat nucleus accumbens: Ultrastructural localization in axon terminals and their relation to dopaminergic afferents. Brain Research. 1988;**444**(2):247-264

[114] Fernandez A, De Ceballos ML, Jenner P, et al. Striatal neuropeptide levels in Parkinson's disease patients. Neuroscience Letters. 1992;**145**(2):171-174

[115] Sivam SP. Dopamine dependent decrease in enkephalin and substance P levels in basal ganglia regions of postmortem parkinsonian brains. Neuropeptides. 1991;**18**(4):201-207

[116] Tirassa P, Schirinzi T, Raspa M, et al. What substance P might tell us about the prognosis and mechanism of Parkinson's disease? Neuroscience and Biobehavioral Reviews. 2021;**131**:899-911

[117] De-Paula VJ, Radanovic M, Diniz BS, et al. Alzheimer's disease. Sub-Cellular Biochemistry. 2012;**65**:329-352

[118] Pákáski M, Kálmán J. Interactions between the amyloid and cholinergic mechanisms in Alzheimer's disease. Neurochemistry International. 2008;**53**(5):103-111

[119] Goldgaber D, Lerman MI, Mcbride OW, et al. Characterization and chromosomal localization of a cDNA encoding brain amyloid of Alzheimer's disease. Science (New York, N.Y.). 1987;**235**(4791):877-880

[120] Glenner GG, Wong CW. Alzheimer's disease and Down's syndrome: Sharing of a unique cerebrovascular amyloid fibril protein. Biochemical and Biophysical Research Communications. 1984;**122**(3):1131-1135

[121] Crystal HA, Davies P. Cortical substance P-like immunoreactivity in cases of Alzheimer's disease and senile dementia of the Alzheimer type. Journal of Neurochemistry. 1982;**38**(6):1781-1784

[122] Bouras C, Vallet PG, Hof PR, et al. Substance P immunoreactivity in Alzheimer disease: A study in cases presenting symmetric or asymmetric cortical atrophy. Alzheimer Disease and Associated Disorders. 1990;**4**(1):24-34

[123] Yankner BA, Duffy LK, Kirschner DA. Neurotrophic and neurotoxic effects of amyloid beta protein: Reversal by tachykinin neuropeptides. Science (New York, N.Y.). 1990;**250**(4978):279-282

[124] Marolda R, Ciotti MT, Matrone C, et al. Substance P activates ADAM9 mRNA expression and induces α-secretase-mediated amyloid precursor protein cleavage. Neuropharmacology. 2012;**62**(5-6):1954-1963

[125] Choi E, Abbott GW. The MiRP2-Kv3.4 potassium channel: Muscling in on Alzheimer's disease. Molecular Pharmacology. 2007;**72**(3):499-501

[126] Severini C, Petrella C, Calissano P. Substance P and Alzheimer's disease: Emerging novel roles. Current Alzheimer Research. 2016;**13**(9):964-972

[127] Ames A 3rd. Energy requirements of CNS cells as related to their function and to their vulnerability to ischemia: A commentary based on studies on retina. Canadian Journal of Physiology and Pharmacology. 1992;**70**(Suppl. S1):58-64

[128] Thoreson WB, Zenisek D. Presynaptic proteins and their roles in visual processing by the retina. Annual Review of Vision Science. 2024;**10**:347-375

[129] Thomas RL, Halim S, Gurudas S, et al. IDF diabetes atlas: A review of studies utilising retinal photography on the global prevalence of diabetes related retinopathy between 2015 and 2018. Diabetes Research and Clinical Practice. 2019;**157**:107840

[130] Ren J, Zhang S, Pan Y, et al. Diabetic retinopathy: Involved cells, biomarkers, and treatments. Frontiers in Pharmacology. 2022;**13**:953691

[131] Troger J, Neyer S, Heufler C, et al. Substance P and vasoactive intestinal polypeptide in the streptozotocin-induced diabetic rat retina. Investigative Ophthalmology & Visual Science. 2001;**42**(5):1045-1050

[132] Kunt T, Forst T, Schmidt S, et al. Serum levels of substance P are decreased in patients with type 1 diabetes. Experimental and Clinical Endocrinology & Diabetes: Official Journal, German Society of Endocrinology [and] German Diabetes Association. 2000;**108**(3):164-167

[133] Sakamoto K, Kuroki T, Sagawa T, et al. Opioid receptor activation is involved in neuroprotection induced by TRPV1 channel activation against excitotoxicity in the rat retina. European Journal of Pharmacology. 2017;**812**:57-63

[134] Yang JH, Guo Z, Zhang T, et al. Restoration of endogenous substance P is associated with inhibition of apoptosis of retinal cells in diabetic rats. Regulatory Peptides. 2013;**187**:12-16

[135] Patrick DM, Leone AK, Shellenberger JJ, et al. Proinflammatory cytokines tumor necrosis factor-alpha and interferon-gamma modulate epithelial barrier function in Madin-Darby canine kidney cells through mitogen activated protein kinase signaling. BMC Physiology. 2006;**6**(2)

[136] Vinores SA, Gadegbeku C, Campochiaro PA, et al. Immunohistochemical localization of blood-retinal barrier breakdown in human diabetics. The American Journal of Pathology. 1989;**134**(2):231-235

[137] Lee D, Hong HS. Substance P alleviates retinal pigment epithelium dysfunction caused by high glucose-induced stress. Life (Basel, Switzerland). 2023;**13**(5):1070-1082

[138] Cowley M, Conway BP, Campochiaro PA, et al. Clinical risk factors for proliferative vitreoretinopathy. Archives of Ophthalmology (Chicago, Ill: 1960). 1989;**107**(8):1147-1151

[139] Ryan SJ. The pathophysiology of proliferative vitreoretinopathy in its management. American Journal of Ophthalmology. 1985;**100**(1):188-193

[140] The classification of retinal detachment with proliferative vitreoretinopathy. Ophthalmology. 1983;**90**(2):121-125

[141] Kieselbach GF, Wiedermann C, Kunze C, et al. Elevated levels of substance P in intraocular fluid in proliferative vitreoretinopathy. Peptides. 1991;**12**(2):275-278

[142] Takahashi E, Nagano O, Ishimoto T, et al. Tumor necrosis factor-alpha regulates transforming growth factor-beta-dependent epithelial-mesenchymal transition by promoting hyaluronan-CD44-moesin interaction. The Journal of Biological Chemistry. 2010;**285**(6):4060-4073

[143] Carrington L, Mcleod D, Boulton M. IL-10 and antibodies to TGF-beta2 and PDGF inhibit RPE-mediated retinal contraction. Investigative Ophthalmology & Visual Science. 2000;**41**(5):1210-1216

[144] D'alessandro A, Cervia D, Catalani E, et al. Protective effects of the neuropeptides PACAP, substance P and the somatostatin analogue octreotide in retinal ischemia: A metabolomic analysis. Molecular BioSystems. 2014;**10**(6):1290-1304

[145] Catalani E, Cervia D, Martini D, et al. Changes in neuronal response to ischemia in retinas with genetic alterations of somatostatin receptor expression. The European Journal of Neuroscience. 2007;**25**(5):1447-1459

[146] Katai N, Yoshimura N. Apoptotic retinal neuronal death by ischemia-reperfusion is executed by two distinct

caspase family proteases. Investigative Ophthalmology & Visual Science. 1999;**40**(11):2697-2705

[147] Rajappa M, Saxena P, Kaur J. Ocular angiogenesis: Mechanisms and recent advances in therapy. Advances in Clinical Chemistry. 2010;**50**:103-121

[148] Tenneti L, Lipton SA. Involvement of activated caspase-3-like proteases in N-methyl-D-aspartate-induced apoptosis in cerebrocortical neurons. Journal of Neurochemistry. 2000;**74**(1):134-142

[149] Jubair S, Li J, Dehlin HM, et al. Substance P induces cardioprotection in ischemia-reperfusion via activation of AKT. American Journal of Physiology Heart and Circulatory Physiology. 2015;**309**(4):H676-H684

[150] Wang L, Wang DH. TRPV1 gene knockout impairs postischemic recovery in isolated perfused heart in mice. Circulation. 2005;**112**(23):3617-3623

[151] Kim DJ, Moon JY, Kim SM, et al. Substance P improves renal ischemia reperfusion injury through modulating immune response. Frontiers in Immunology. 2020;**11**:600

[152] Engelmann K, Valtink M. RPE cell cultivation. Graefe's Archive for Clinical and Experimental Ophthalmology = Albrecht von Graefes Archiv fur klinische und experimentelle Ophthalmologie. 2004;**242**(1):65-67

[153] Sparrow JR, Hicks D, Hamel CP. The retinal pigment epithelium in health and disease. Current Molecular Medicine. 2010;**10**(9):802-823

[154] Harman D. The aging process. Proceedings of the National Academy of Sciences of the United States of America. 1981;**78**(11):7124-7128

[155] Fanjul-Moles ML, López-Riquelme GO. Relationship between oxidative stress, circadian rhythms, and AMD. Oxidative Medicine and Cellular Longevity. 2016;**2016**:7420637

[156] Binder S, Stanzel BV, Krebs I, et al. Transplantation of the RPE in AMD. Progress in Retinal and Eye Research. 2007;**26**(5):516-554

[157] Schnabolk G. Systemic inflammatory disease and AMD comorbidity. Advances in Experimental Medicine and Biology. 2019;**1185**:27-31

[158] Hong HS, Son Y. Substance P ameliorates collagen II-induced arthritis in mice via suppression of the inflammatory response. Biochemical and Biophysical Research Communications. 2014;**453**(1):179-184

[159] Jiang MH, Chung E, Chi GF, et al. Substance P induces M2-type macrophages after spinal cord injury. Neuroreport. 2012;**23**(13):786-792

[160] Hong HS, Kim S, Nam S, et al. Effect of substance P on recovery from laser-induced retinal degeneration. Wound Repair and Regeneration: Official Publication of the Wound Healing Society [and] the European Tissue Repair Society. 2015;**23**(2):268-277

[161] Fan JB, Yuan K, Zhu XH, et al. Neuroligin-3 activates Akt-dependent Nrf2 cascade to protect osteoblasts from oxidative stress. Free Radical Biology & Medicine. 2023;**208**:807-819

[162] Klettner A. Oxidative stress induced cellular signaling in RPE cells. Frontiers in Bioscience (Scholar Edition). 2012;**4**(2):392-411

[163] Baek SM, Yu SY, Son Y, et al. Substance P promotes the recovery of oxidative stress-damaged retinal

pigmented epithelial cells by modulating Akt/GSK-3β signaling. Molecular Vision. 2016;**22**:1015-1023

[164] Ziche M, Morbidelli L, Masini E, et al. Nitric oxide mediates angiogenesis in vivo and endothelial cell growth and migration in vitro promoted by substance P. The Journal of Clinical Investigation. 1994;**94**(5):2036-2044

[165] Shaik-Dasthagirisaheb YB, Varvara G, Murmura G, et al. Vascular endothelial growth factor (VEGF), mast cells and inflammation. International Journal of Immunopathology and Pharmacology. 2013;**26**(2):327-335

[166] Katsanos GS, Anogeianaki A, Orso C, et al. Impact of substance P on cellular immunity. Journal of Biological Regulators and Homeostatic Agents. 2008;**22**(2):93-98

[167] Lee IG, Chae SL, Kim JC. Involvement of circulating endothelial progenitor cells and vasculogenic factors in the pathogenesis of diabetic retinopathy. Eye (London, England). 2006;**20**(5):546-552

[168] Cunin P, Caillon A, Corvaisier M, et al. The tachykinins substance P and hemokinin-1 favor the generation of human memory Th17 cells by inducing IL-1β, IL-23, and TNF-like 1A expression by monocytes. Journal of Immunology. 2011;**186**(7):4175-4182

[169] De Felipe C, Herrero JF, O'brien JA, et al. Altered nociception, analgesia and aggression in mice lacking the receptor for substance P. Nature. 1998;**392**(6674):394-397

[170] Bozic CR, Lu B, Höpken UE, et al. Neurogenic amplification of immune complex inflammation. Science (New York, N.Y.). 1996;**273**(5282):1722-1725

[171] Neumann S, Doubell TP, Leslie T, et al. Inflammatory pain hypersensitivity mediated by phenotypic switch in myelinated primary sensory neurons. Nature. 1996;**384**(6607):360-364

[172] Noguchi K, Ruda MA. Gene regulation in an ascending nociceptive pathway: Inflammation-induced increase in preprotachykinin mRNA in rat lamina I spinal projection neurons. The Journal of Neuroscience. 1992;**12**(7):2563-2572

[173] Rubinstein M, Mogil JS, Japón M, et al. Absence of opioid stress-induced analgesia in mice lacking beta-endorphin by site-directed mutagenesis. Proceedings of the National Academy of Sciences of the United States of America. 1996;**93**(9):3995-4000

[174] Marek P, Mogil JS, Sternberg WF, et al. N-methyl-D-aspartic acid (NMDA) receptor antagonist MK-801 blocks non-opioid stress-induced analgesia. II. Comparison across three swim-stress paradigms in selectively bred mice. Brain Research. 1992;**578**(1-2):197-203

[175] Vanderah TW, Wild KD, Takemori AE, et al. Mediation of swim-stress antinociception by the opioid delta 2 receptor in the mouse. The Journal of Pharmacology and Experimental Therapeutics. 1992;**262**(1):190-197

[176] Jessell TM, Iversen LL. Opiate analgesics inhibit substance P release from rat trigeminal nucleus. Nature. 1977;**268**(5620):549-551

[177] Thornton E, Vink R. Treatment with a substance P receptor antagonist is neuroprotective in the intrastriatal 6-hydroxydopamine model of early Parkinson's disease. PLoS One. 2012;**7**(4):e34138

[178] Kowall NW, Quigley BJ Jr, Krause JE, et al. Substance P and

substance P receptor histochemistry in human neurodegenerative diseases. Regulatory Peptides. 1993;**46**(1-2):174-185

[179] Barker R, Larner A. Substance P and multiple sclerosis. Medical Hypotheses. 1992;**37**(1):40-43

[180] Reid MS, Hökfelt T, Herrera-Marschitz M, et al. Intranigral substance P stimulation of striatal dopamine release is inhibited by spantide II: A new tachykinin antagonist without apparent neurotoxicity. Brain Research. 1990;**532**(1-2):175-181

[181] Gao X, Bayraktutan U. Substance P reversibly compromises the integrity and function of blood-brain barrier. Peptides. 2023;**167**:171048

[182] Safwat A, Helmy A, Gupta A. The role of Substance P within traumatic brain injury and implications for therapy. Journal of Neurotrauma. 2023;**40**(15-16):1567-1583

[183] Lewis KM, Turner RJ, Vink R. Blocking neurogenic inflammation for the treatment of acute disorders of the central nervous system. International Journal of Inflammation. 2013;**2013**:578480

[184] Hertz L, Mcfarlin DE, Waksman BH. Astrocytes: Auxiliary cells for immune responses in the central nervous system? Immunology Today. 1990;**11**(8):265-268

[185] Compston A, Scolding N, Wren D, et al. The pathogenesis of demyelinating disease: Insights from cell biology. Trends in Neurosciences. 1991;**14**(5):175-182

[186] Cramer H, Rösler N, Rissler K, et al. Cerebrospinal fluid immunoreactive substance P and somatostatin in neurological patients with peripheral and spinal cord disease. Neuropeptides. 1988;**12**(3):119-124

[187] Sharma HS, Nyberg F, Olsson Y, et al. Alteration of substance P after trauma to the spinal cord: An experimental study in the rat. Neuroscience. 1990;**38**(1):205-212

[188] Naftchi NE, Abrahams SJ, St. Paul HM, et al. Localization and changes of substance P in spinal cord of paraplegic cats. Brain Research. 1978;**153**(3):507-513

[189] Faden AI, Jacobs TP, Helke CJ. Changes in substance P and somatostatin in the spinal cord after traumatic spinal injury in the rat. Neuropeptides. 1985;**6**(3):215-225

[190] Vita G, Haun CK, Hawkins EF, et al. Effects of experimental spinal cord transection on substance P receptors: A quantitative autoradiography study. Neuropeptides. 1990;**17**(3):147-153

[191] Preston E, Sutherland G, Finsten A. Three openings of the blood-brain barrier produced by forebrain ischemia in the rat. Neuroscience Letters. 1993;**149**(1):75-78

[192] Turner RJ, Helps SC, Thornton E, et al. A substance P antagonist improves outcome when administered 4 h after onset of ischaemic stroke. Brain Research. 2011;**1393**:84-90

[193] Yu Z, Cheng G, Huang X, et al. Neurokinin-1 receptor antagonist SR140333: A novel type of drug to treat cerebral ischemia. Neuroreport. 1997;**8**(9-10):2117-2119

[194] Turner RJ, Vink R. Combined tissue plasminogen activator and an NK1 tachykinin receptor antagonist: An effective treatment for reperfusion injury following acute ischemic stroke in rats. Neuroscience. 2012;**220**:1-10

[195] Vink R, Van Den Heuvel C. Substance P antagonists as a therapeutic approach to improving outcome following traumatic brain injury. Neurotherapeutics. 2010;**7**(1):74-80

[196] He H, Kuriyan AE, Su CW, et al. Inhibition of proliferation and epithelial mesenchymal transition in retinal pigment epithelial cells by heavy chain-Hyaluronan/Pentraxin 3. Scientific Reports. 2017;**7**:43736

[197] Jorge R, Oyamaguchi EK, Cardillo JA, et al. Intravitreal injection of dispase causes retinal hemorrhages in rabbit and human eyes. Current Eye Research. 2003;**26**(2):107-112

[198] Pastor JC, De La Rúa ER, Martín F. Proliferative vitreoretinopathy: Risk factors and pathobiology. Progress in Retinal and Eye Research. 2002;**21**(1):127-144

[199] Isiksoy S, Basmak H, Kasapoglu Dundar E, et al. Expression of proteins associated with cell-matrix adhesion in proliferative vitreoretinopathy designed by Dispase model. European Journal of Ophthalmology. 2007;**17**(1):89-103

[200] Frenzel EM, Neely KA, Walsh AW, et al. A new model of proliferative vitreoretinopathy. Investigative Ophthalmology & Visual Science. 1998;**39**(11):2157-2164

[201] Sheridan CM, Occleston NL, Hiscott P, et al. Matrix metalloproteinases: A role in the contraction of vitreo-retinal scar tissue. The American Journal of Pathology. 2001;**159**(4):1555-1566

[202] Zhu XJ, Wolff D, Zhang KK, et al. Molecular inflammation in the contralateral eye after cataract surgery in the first eye. Investigative Ophthalmology & Visual Science. 2015;**56**(9):5566-5573

[203] Zhang Y, Du Y, Jiang Y, et al. Effects of pranoprofen on aqueous humor monocyte chemoattractant Protein-1 level and pain relief during second-eye cataract surgery. Frontiers in Pharmacology. 2018;**9**:783

[204] Spitsin S, Meshki J, Winters A, et al. Substance P-mediated chemokine production promotes monocyte migration. Journal of Leukocyte Biology. 2017;**101**(4):967-973

[205] Fang K, Law IKM, Padua D, et al. MicroRNA-31-3p is involved in Substance P (SP)-associated inflammation in human colonic epithelial cells and experimental colitis. The American Journal of Pathology. 2018;**188**(3):586-599

[206] Hayashi Y, Kajimoto K, Iida S, et al. DNA microarray analysis of whole blood cells and insulin-sensitive tissues reveals the usefulness of blood RNA profiling as a source of markers for predicting type 2 diabetes. Biological & Pharmaceutical Bulletin. 2010;**33**(6):1033-1042

[207] Yang JH, Kwak HW, Kim TG, et al. Retinal neurodegeneration in type II diabetic Otsuka long-Evans Tokushima fatty rats. Investigative Ophthalmology & Visual Science. 2013;**54**(6):3844-3851

[208] Kim KS, Oh DH, Kim JY, et al. Taurine ameliorates hyperglycemia and dyslipidemia by reducing insulin resistance and leptin level in Otsuka long-Evans Tokushima fatty (OLETF) rats with long-term diabetes. Experimental & Molecular Medicine. 2012;**44**(11):665-673

[209] Yin MJ, Yamamoto Y, Gaynor RB. The anti-inflammatory agents aspirin and salicylate inhibit the activity of I(kappa)B kinase-beta. Nature. 1998;**396**(6706):77-80

[210] Yuan M, Konstantopoulos N, Lee J, et al. Reversal of obesity- and diet-induced insulin resistance with salicylates or targeted disruption of Ikkbeta. Science. 2001;**293**(5535):1673-1677

[211] Petrella RJ, Blouin J, Davies B, et al. Prevalence, demographics, and treatment characteristics of visual impairment due to diabetic macular Edema in a representative Canadian cohort. Journal of Ophthalmology. 2012;**2012**:159167

[212] Laha B, Stafford BK, Huberman AD. Regenerating optic pathways from the eye to the brain. Science. 2017;**356**(6342):1031-1034

[213] Kugler M, Schlecht A, Fuchshofer R, et al. Heterozygous modulation of TGF-β signaling does not influence Müller glia cell reactivity or proliferation following NMDA-induced damage. Histochemistry and Cell Biology. 2015;**144**(5):443-455

[214] Sheridan CM, Rice D, Hiscott PS, et al. The presence of AC133-positive cells suggests a possible role of endothelial progenitor cells in the formation of choroidal neovascularization. Investigative Ophthalmology & Visual Science. 2006;**47**(4):1642-1645

[215] Harris JR, Brown GA, Jorgensen M, et al. Bone marrow-derived cells home to and regenerate retinal pigment epithelium after injury. Investigative Ophthalmology & Visual Science. 2006;**47**(5):2108-2113

[216] Asahara T, Masuda H, Takahashi T, et al. Bone marrow origin of endothelial progenitor cells responsible for postnatal vasculogenesis in physiological and pathological neovascularization. Circulation Research. 1999;**85**(3):221-228

[217] Asahara T, Takahashi T, Masuda H, et al. VEGF contributes to postnatal neovascularization by mobilizing bone marrow-derived endothelial progenitor cells. The EMBO Journal. 1999;**18**(14):3964-3972

Chapter 5

Functional Neurological Disorder: A Neurobiological Perspective on Maladaptive Plasticity

Ioannis Mavroudis, Foivos Petrides, Katerina Franekova, Alin Ciobica and Dimitrios Kazis

Abstract

Functional Neurological Disorder (FND) is a common, often misunderstood condition at the intersection of neurology and psychiatry. It presents with motor, sensory, cognitive, and seizure-like symptoms that are not consistent with known neurological diseases. Historically viewed as psychogenic, FND is now understood as a disorder of brain network dysfunction and maladaptive neuroplasticity, rather than structural pathology. Recent studies frame FND as a dynamic condition involving disrupted communication across sensorimotor, limbic, and cognitive control circuits. Central features include impaired self-agency, abnormal predictive coding, and disrupted emotion-motor integration. Contemporary models, drawing from Bayesian inference and network neuroscience, propose that symptoms result from the brain's misinterpretation of internal signals, influenced by expectation and attention. Neuroimaging highlights dysfunction in regions such as the temporoparietal junction, limbic-prefrontal pathways, and networks like the salience and default mode networks. These abnormalities help explain impaired volitional control and symptom persistence. Stress, trauma, and suggestion may reinforce symptoms through mechanisms like fear learning, heightened interoceptive awareness, and maladaptive synaptic changes. Diagnosis relies on positive clinical signs—such as Hoover's sign and tremor entrainment—rather than exclusion of disease. FND frequently coexists with psychiatric or neurological conditions. Treatment includes psychoeducation, physiotherapy, cognitive-behavioral therapy (CBT), and, in some cases, neuromodulation techniques like transcranial magnetic stimulation (TMS). Encouragingly, interventions like CBT and physiotherapy have shown measurable improvements in brain connectivity and motor function, supporting the reversible nature of FND. Understanding FND as a neurobiologically grounded disorder fosters effective, compassionate care and opens pathways to the targeted therapies.

Keywords: functional neurological disorder (FND), brain network dysfunction, maladaptive neuroplasticity, predictive coding, sensorimotor integration, bayesian inference, neuroimaging biomarkers

1. Introduction

Functional Neurological Disorder (FND), historically referred to as conversion disorder, is a condition characterized by neurological symptoms—such as motor deficits, non-epileptic seizures, or sensory disturbances—that are incompatible with recognized disease processes. While long considered purely psychogenic, modern neurobiological research has reframed FND as a disorder of aberrant brain network function and plasticity [1, 2].

FND lies at the intersection of neurology and psychiatry, involving dysfunctional connectivity between sensorimotor, limbic, and cognitive control regions. Neuroimaging studies consistently reveal alterations in brain networks subserving self-agency, emotional regulation, and interoception, challenging the Cartesian mind–body split and offering a unified model rooted in network neuroscience [3, 4].

Critically, FND is not a fixed structural lesion but a dynamic brain state shaped by maladaptive plasticity. Aberrant neuroplastic mechanisms—potentially initiated by stress, trauma, illness, or suggestion—may lead to reinforced symptom circuits, akin to learned behaviors or memory traces. This framework places synaptic plasticity at the core of FND pathophysiology and opens avenues for biologically informed interventions.

The clinical burden of FND is substantial. It represents one of the most common diagnoses in outpatient neurology clinics, yet it is frequently misunderstood and stigmatized. Misdiagnosis, delayed care, and inappropriate testing or treatment contribute to patient distress and system inefficiency [5, 6].

In this chapter, we present a comprehensive overview of FND through the lens of maladaptive plasticity and network dysfunction. We synthesize evidence from neuroimaging, electrophysiology, neuropsychology, and emerging translational models to illuminate how the brain's inherent capacity for change—normally a substrate for learning and recovery—can lead to disabling symptoms in the absence of structural pathology. We also explore therapeutic implications, including targeted rehabilitation, neuromodulation, and psychoeducational models that seek to rewire dysfunctional circuits and restore agency.

2. Pathophysiology and neurocircuitry of FND

Functional Neurological Disorder (FND) is increasingly recognized as a disorder of impaired self-agency, dysfunctional prediction error signaling, and maladaptive interactions between cognitive, motor, and emotional systems (**Figure 1**). While symptoms mimic those seen in structural neurological disease, FND is underpinned by abnormal functional integration and plasticity rather than fixed lesions [7].

2.1 Cortico-subcortical network disruption

Modern neuroimaging consistently reveals aberrant connectivity across key cortico-subcortical networks in FND, including:

- Sensorimotor circuits: Studies have shown hypoactivation in primary motor and supplementary motor areas during movement attempts in patients with functional weakness or tremor. Simultaneously, increased activity in limbic areas such as the amygdala and anterior insula suggests emotional interference with motor output.

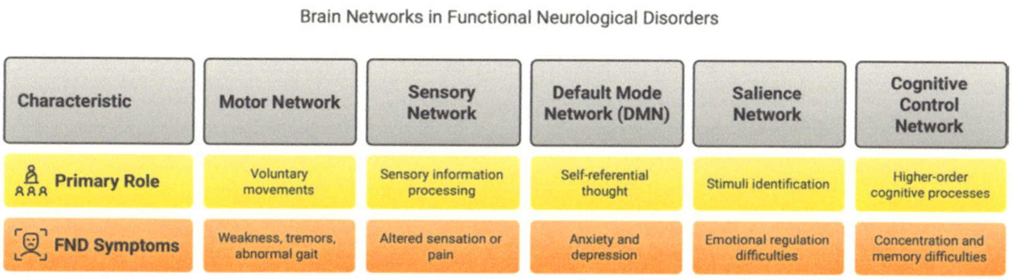

Figure 1.
Cerebral Network Alterations in Functional Neurological Disorder (FND): This figure illustrates disrupted connectivity in cortico-subcortical loops, emphasizing the role of sensorimotor, limbic, and salience networks in generating functional symptoms. It visualizes the interplay between impaired self-agency, heightened emotional salience, and network-level inefficiency.

- Default Mode Network (DMN): Altered DMN coherence is observed in patients with dissociative or seizure-like symptoms, pointing to instability in self-referential processing and internal narrative construction [3].

- Salience and executive networks: Disruptions here may impair top-down attentional control and enhance symptom-focused attention, consistent with the strong influence of expectation and suggestibility in FND [8].

These alterations form the basis of functional disconnection models, in which symptoms arise from network-level inefficiency in integrating volitional intent with sensory feedback and emotional context.

2.2 The role of self-agency and prediction error

FND is increasingly framed as a disorder of self-agency, wherein patients experience actions or sensations as involuntary despite being internally generated. This aligns with predictive coding theories, which suggest that the brain continuously generates predictions about incoming sensory input. When there is a mismatch (prediction error), these are normally resolved via attention or behavior updates.

In FND, however, high-level priors (expectations) dominate perception and override contradictory bottom-up signals, leading to the experience of involuntariness [2, 7]. For instance, a patient may unconsciously anticipate weakness or seizure, and that expectation shapes motor output accordingly—even in the absence of structural pathology.

This model is supported by findings of abnormal temporoparietal junction (TPJ) activity, a key hub for distinguishing self-generated from external stimuli. Dysfunction in this area may contribute to impaired awareness of agency, as observed in both motor and sensory subtypes of FND [9].

2.3 Emotional dysregulation and limbic hyperactivity

Emotional processes are not merely comorbid but integral to FND pathophysiology. Limbic structures—including the amygdala, anterior cingulate cortex (ACC), and insula—show increased activation and connectivity in patients with functional symptoms, particularly in response to emotionally salient stimuli [10].

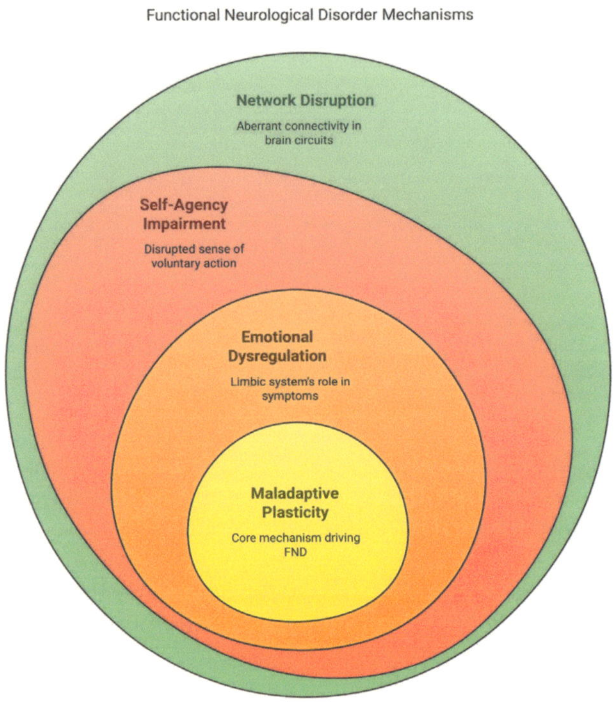

Figure 2.
This nested diagram illustrates key mechanisms in Functional Neurological Disorder (FND), from outer network disruption to core maladaptive plasticity. Each layer represents a contributing domain, with plasticity shaping symptoms through disrupted agency, emotion, and connectivity. The model emphasizes FND as a disorder of dynamic, reversible brain network dysfunction.

This suggests that emotional salience is improperly weighted, leading to somatic symptom expression and inappropriate limbic-motor coupling. Functional symptoms may thus reflect overlearned emotional responses reenacted through motor or sensory channels, driven by heightened limbic influence and insufficient executive inhibition.

2.4 Maladaptive plasticity and memory mechanisms

There is growing evidence that FND symptoms reflect a form of maladaptive plasticity, where prior traumatic, suggestive, or emotionally charged experiences are "learned" into sensorimotor or interoceptive networks. This may involve mechanisms akin to Hebbian learning, where circuits activated together during high salience events become abnormally reinforced (**Figure 2**).

Analogies have been drawn between FND and fear memory consolidation, suggesting that functional symptoms may be engrained like trauma responses, but expressed *via* movement or sensation rather than affect alone [11]. Persistent symptoms might therefore reflect long-term potentiation (LTP)-like synaptic changes in dysfunctional circuits, rather than fleeting psychological stressors.

2.5 Summary of neural mechanisms

See (**Table 1**).

Domain	Key brain structures	Abnormal findings
Self-agency	Temporoparietal junction, SMA	Disrupted intention-action mapping, altered sense of ownership
Emotion-motor integration	Amygdala, insula, anterior cingulate cortex	Limbic hyperactivity linked to motor inhibition
Executive control	Dorsolateral prefrontal cortex, ACC	Impaired top-down regulation of attention and inhibition
Sensory processing	Primary somatosensory cortex, insula	Abnormal gain on interoceptive inputs
Motor output	SMA, M1, basal ganglia	Hypoactivation during voluntary movement

Table 1.
Neural domains and associated abnormalities in FND: This table summarizes the core neural domains implicated in FND, including disrupted self-agency, emotion-motor integration, sensory processing, executive control, and motor output. It maps key brain structures to the corresponding abnormal findings observed in neuroimaging and electrophysiological studies.

3. Clinical features and diagnostic challenges

Functional Neurological Disorder (FND) presents a spectrum of neurological symptoms that appear clinically inconsistent or incongruent with recognized structural disease yet are genuine, disabling, and often persistent. The wide range of presentations and overlap with both neurological and psychiatric disorders contribute to its under-recognition, diagnostic delay, and therapeutic uncertainty [6, 12].

3.1 Core clinical presentations

Clinicians must differentiate functional symptoms from organic counterparts by emphasizing inconsistency across examinations, presence of positive signs, and their sensitivity to attention and context.

The diagnosis of FND is based on positive clinical signs, not exclusion. Current diagnostic approaches emphasize features that distinguish FND from mimics, such as inconsistency and incongruence [1]. *Rather than relying solely on the absence of structural abnormalities, clinicians identify FND through observable signs that directly demonstrate the mismatch between symptoms and known neurological patterns. This positive approach enhances diagnostic clarity and facilitates therapeutic engagement.*

3.1.1 Motor symptoms

Motor symptoms are among the most frequent presentations of FND, typically manifesting as weakness, abnormal movements, or gait disturbance. These symptoms often emerge abruptly and fluctuate in intensity, defying the expected progression of organic neurological disorders.

- Functional weakness or paralysis: Often characterized by sudden onset, variability over time, and specific signs such as Hoover's sign or abductor sign [13]. Unlike true paresis due to structural lesions, functional weakness demonstrates internally inconsistent findings, such as normal power during automatic tasks and weakness during voluntary movement.

- Tremor, dystonia, gait disturbance: Functional movement disorders frequently show entrainment, distractibility, and variability—features rarely seen in organic conditions [14]. *For example, a functional tremor may vanish during contralateral motor tasks, while organic tremors typically persist regardless of attention or distraction.*

Functional gait patterns may appear bizarre but are often associated with normal balance, absence of falls, and exaggerated slowness or leg stiffness, which improve when attention is shifted away from walking. Such features strongly favor a functional origin over neurodegenerative causes.

3.1.2 Functional seizures (PNES)

- Psychogenic non-epileptic seizures (PNES) may resemble tonic–clonic or focal seizures but typically lack stereotypy, have prolonged duration, asynchronous movements, and are not associated with ictal EEG changes [15]. *In contrast to epilepsy, PNES episodes often occur in emotionally charged contexts, are more frequent when witnessed, and tend to resist antiepileptic medication. Clinical indicators such as long duration, side-to-side head movements, or closed eyes during episodes are helpful in distinguishing PNES from epileptic seizures.*

3.1.3 Sensory and speech symptoms

- *Functional sensory loss* may present in nonanatomical distributions (e.g., sharply demarcated hemianesthesia at the midline) or with internal inconsistencies, such as preserved sensation during distraction or mismatch with reflex integrity. *Examiners often find that tactile or pinprick responses fluctuate within the same exam, unlike the stable deficits seen in peripheral or central sensory lesions.*

- *Functional dysphonia, aphonia, or stuttering* can appear suddenly and are often triggered by stress or trauma. They may occur in isolation or alongside other functional symptoms [16]. *These speech abnormalities usually preserve automatic speech (e.g., singing or shouting), which is atypical for organic causes and indicative of a functional mechanism.*

3.1.4 Functional cognitive disorder (FCD)

- FCD is increasingly recognized as a subtype of FND involving self-reported cognitive deficits (e.g., memory, concentration), often with heightened health anxiety and internal inconsistency during neuropsychological testing [17]. *A hallmark of FCD is the discrepancy between perceived impairment and test results, with common patterns including poor performance on simple tasks but normal function on more demanding ones. FCD may coexist with anxiety, depression, or post-concussion symptoms, and often reflects heightened self-monitoring and health anxiety rather than progressive cognitive decline.*

3.2 Diagnostic criteria and frameworks

Diagnosis is clinical, based on history and examination, not on exclusion of pathology. The DSM-5 criteria specify the requirement for at least one symptom of altered voluntary motor or sensory function, with evidence of incompatibility between the symptom and recognized neurological conditions [18].

Key diagnostic clues include:

- Positive signs (e.g., Hoover's sign, tremor entrainment).
- Variability and context-dependence.
- Nonanatomical distribution of symptoms.
- Lack of organic explanation despite extensive workup.

Neuroimaging and electrophysiological studies are often used to support rather than confirm the diagnosis, helping to reassure patients and rule out mimics.

3.3 Common diagnostic pitfalls

- Misattribution to malingering or feigning: FND symptoms are not under voluntary control, and mislabeling patients can erode trust and delay care.
- Delayed recognition: Patients often undergo multiple referrals and investigations before diagnosis, increasing costs and emotional burden.
- Overdiagnosis risk exists, especially when positive signs are not carefully evaluated, or comorbidities are missed.

3.4 Psychiatric comorbidity and stigma

While psychiatric comorbidity—particularly anxiety, depression, trauma history, and dissociation—is common in FND, it is not required for diagnosis [19]. Overemphasis on psychological causation can perpetuate the false dichotomy between "real" and "psychogenic" illness.

Stigma remains a major challenge, both from healthcare providers and the public. Reframing FND as a brain-based disorder of network dysfunction and maladaptive plasticity is key to reducing stigma and improving care.

3.5 Functional overlay and diagnostic coexistence

FND can coexist with structural or neurodegenerative disorders. Functional overlay in conditions such as multiple sclerosis, epilepsy, Parkinson's disease, or TBI is increasingly recognized, requiring careful diagnostic skill to distinguish and manage each component appropriately [20].

4. Neuroplasticity and learning mechanisms in FND

Functional Neurological Disorder (FND) can be conceptualized as a disorder of maladaptive plasticity—the brain's capacity to adapt to experience in ways that, under certain conditions, reinforce dysfunctional patterns of perception, movement, and cognition. This view unites FND with other neurobehavioral conditions where abnormal learning, attentional bias, and synaptic reinforcement contribute to persistent symptoms [7, 21].

4.1 Experience-dependent plasticity and symptom formation

Plasticity refers to the brain's ability to modify its structure and function in response to internal or external stimuli. In FND, highly salient experiences, including illness, trauma, suggestion, or expectation, may become embedded in sensorimotor networks via Hebbian learning processes—"cells that fire together wire together" [22].

For instance, a transient episode of dissociation or injury-induced weakness may become reinforced through repeated attention, avoidance, and emotional valence. This can lead to "learned nonuse", where voluntary control is suppressed not by damage, but by maladaptive cortical inhibition and synaptic downregulation [23].

4.2 Aberrant reinforcement and memory encoding

FND symptoms can be encoded through non-declarative memory systems, such as procedural or emotional memory. As with fear conditioning or habit formation, repetition of emotionally charged motor responses may strengthen dysfunctional circuits, particularly when paired with avoidance learning or perceived threat [4, 11].

Neuroimaging supports this model. Enhanced amygdala-SMA connectivity has been observed in patients with functional motor symptoms, suggesting emotion-motor coupling may act as a plasticity driver [9]. Similarly, default mode and salience network disruptions may facilitate symptom-focused attention and persistence through feedback loops.

4.3 Cortical inhibition and network reweighting

FND is associated with abnormal inhibitory control and inter-regional communication, particularly in networks involved in self-agency and volition. Transcranial magnetic stimulation (TMS) studies show reduced cortical excitability and suppression of motor potentials, especially in voluntary but not reflexive movement tasks [24].

This suggests that top-down inhibition from prefrontal regions may suppress motor execution, not through paralysis, but through circuit-level gating. Over time, these patterns may be reweighted through synaptic depression or altered gain control, particularly in circuits involving the SMA, anterior cingulate, and temporoparietal junction.

4.4 Interoception, attention, and predictive coding

Interoceptive awareness—the brain's perception of internal bodily states—is often distorted in FND, and this has plastic implications. Heightened interoceptive precision (over-weighted bodily signals) or distorted priors (expectations) may alter network gain in the insula, anterior cingulate, and brainstem nuclei, reinforcing symptoms through attentional salience [25].

Over time, these attentional shifts may create trait-like neuroplastic changes, akin to those observed in anxiety and chronic pain syndromes, where network reorganization supports ongoing symptom vigilance, suppression of volition, and enhanced somatic awareness [26].

Plastic process	Adaptive outcome	Maladaptive outcome (FND)
Motor learning	Skill acquisition	Learned motor inhibition, functional weakness
Emotional conditioning	Appropriate fear response	Amplified symptom expression, PNES
Interoceptive tuning	Improved body awareness	Heightened symptom vigilance, dissociation
Cortical reweighting	Efficient sensorimotor integration	Incongruent movement planning and execution

Table 2.
Maladaptive versus adaptive plasticity in FND: This table contrasts typical adaptive outcomes of neural plasticity (e.g., skill acquisition or improved awareness) with maladaptive expressions seen in FND, such as learned motor inhibition or heightened symptom vigilance. It highlights how core plastic processes can yield either functional or dysfunctional results depending on context and reinforcement.

4.5 Maladaptive vs. adaptive plasticity: A clinical continuum

Plasticity in FND is not inherently pathological; it reflects the brain's capacity to adapt to internal models. What distinguishes maladaptive from adaptive plasticity is the functional outcome (**Table 2**). For instance:

Rehabilitation in FND thus seeks not to erase plasticity but to redirect it toward functional patterns—a goal achieved through therapy, retraining, and neuromodulation.

5. Therapeutic approaches and circuit-based interventions

A modern understanding of FND as a disorder of brain network dysregulation and maladaptive plasticity has reshaped treatment from psychodynamic and exclusion-based models toward targeted, interdisciplinary interventions. The goal is to restore function by leveraging the brain's capacity for adaptive plasticity, promoting reorganization of dysfunctional circuits through behavioral, cognitive, and neuromodulatory strategies [27].

5.1 Psychoeducation and diagnostic delivery

Effective treatment begins with how the diagnosis is communicated. Studies show that when clinicians explain FND as a brain-based disorder with identifiable clinical features (e.g., Hoover's sign), patient acceptance improves [13].

Key principles:

- Use clear, non-dualistic language (e.g., "real and treatable," "software not hardware").
- Emphasize positive diagnostic signs over exclusion of disease.
- Provide written or video resources to reinforce understanding [28].

This "diagnosis-as-treatment" model activates reappraisal circuits and may initiate neuroplastic shifts even before formal therapy begins.

5.2 Physiotherapy and sensorimotor retraining

Functional motor symptoms (e.g., weakness, tremor, gait disturbances) respond well to specialist physiotherapy designed to restore automaticity and reduce symptom-focused attention [29].

Features of effective physiotherapy:

- Focus on normal movement patterns rather than pathology.
- Use of distraction, dual-tasking, or guided imagery to bypass dysfunctional networks.
- Re-engagement of motor circuits through implicit learning, restoring SMA and M1 activation.

Randomized trials show improved mobility, strength, and quality of life with this approach, often more effectively than generic rehabilitation [30].

5.3 Cognitive-Behavioral therapy (CBT) and emotional regulation

CBT is the most evidence-supported psychotherapy for FND, particularly for functional seizures and sensory symptoms [31]. Its targets include:

- Symptom-related fear and avoidance (e.g., catastrophic beliefs about seizures).
- Attentional bias and misattribution (e.g., interpreting bodily signals as dangerous).
- Emotional dysregulation and trauma processing when relevant.

CBT may alter network dynamics by modulating limbic-prefrontal connectivity, reducing hypervigilance, and fostering top-down inhibitory control.

Emerging modalities such as Acceptance and Commitment Therapy (ACT) and interoceptive retraining further enrich the cognitive-affective toolbox.

5.4 Multidisciplinary and inpatient programs

Complex or refractory cases often require integrated neurorehabilitation, involving:

- Neurologists, physiotherapists, psychologists, occupational therapists, and speech/language therapists.
- Group and individual formats combining motor, cognitive, and emotional retraining.

Such programs achieve neuroplastic reeducation by delivering coordinated stimuli across multiple circuits. Inpatient units report meaningful improvements in function and reduced healthcare utilization [32].

5.5 Neuromodulation and experimental interventions

Given FND's basis in network dysregulation, brain stimulation techniques are under investigation:

- Transcranial magnetic stimulation (TMS) to the motor cortex or dorsolateral prefrontal cortex shows promise in restoring voluntary movement and reducing motor symptoms [24, 33].
- tDCS (transcranial direct current stimulation) may modulate network excitability and interoceptive gain in patients with functional seizures or motor deficits.
- Neurofeedback and real-time fMRI offer personalized feedback to normalize agency and emotional circuits, though data are preliminary [34].

These interventions aim to recalibrate dysfunctional circuits through externally guided plasticity, often in conjunction with behavioral therapies.

5.6 Long-term management and prognosis

FND prognosis varies. Positive predictors include:

- Early diagnosis and explanation.
- Presence of positive signs.
- Patient engagement and insight.
- Absence of entrenched secondary gain or chronic disability.

Entrenched maladaptive learning, comorbid affective or personality disorders, or socioeconomic barriers may drive persistent symptoms. In such cases, long-term supportive care, psychiatric collaboration, and social interventions become essential.

6. Conclusion

Functional Neurological Disorder (FND) exemplifies the complex interplay between neurobiology, cognition, emotion, and behavior. Once relegated to the margins of neurology as a psychogenic curiosity, FND is now understood as a brain-based condition rooted in network dysfunction, impaired self-agency, and maladaptive neuroplasticity.

Advances in neuroimaging, electrophysiology, and cognitive neuroscience have elucidated key features of FND pathophysiology: disruption of sensorimotor and limbic-prefrontal circuits, aberrant predictive coding, impaired top-down control, and enhanced emotional-motor coupling. Crucially, these mechanisms do not reflect fixed damage but reversible maladaptations, positioning FND as a disorder of dynamic plasticity rather than degeneration.

Clinically, FND presents with a rich array of motor, sensory, cognitive, and seizure-like symptoms. Positive signs—such as variability, entrainment, and incongruence—are central to diagnosis and distinguish FND from malingering or structural disease. Coexisting psychiatric symptoms are common but not universal and must be approached with sensitivity to avoid stigmatization.

Treatment of FND has evolved into a multidisciplinary, circuit-based approach, combining neurologically informed explanation, physiotherapy, cognitive-behavioral strategies, and—where indicated—neuromodulation. These therapies aim not simply to manage symptoms but to retrain dysfunctional circuits, leveraging the brain's capacity for recovery and reorganization.

The study of FND not only improves outcomes for a long-neglected patient group but also offers broader insights into how perception, agency, emotion, and volition are constructed in the brain. In this light, FND serves as a model condition for exploring plasticity gone awry, underscoring the need for ongoing integration of neuroscience, psychology, and compassionate care.

Author details

Ioannis Mavroudis[1,2,3]*, Foivos Petrides[2], Katerina Franekova[3], Alin Ciobica[4,5,6,7] and Dimitrios Kazis[2]

1 Department of Neuroscience, Leeds Teaching Hospitals, UK

2 Third Department of Neurology, Aristotle University of Thessaloniki, Greece

3 School of Medicine, University of Leeds, Leeds, UK

4 Department of Biology, Faculty of Biology, Alexandru Ioan Cuza University of Iasi, Iasi, Romania

5 Center of Biomedical Research, Romanian Academy, Iasi Branch, Iasi, Romania

6 Academy of Romanian Scientists, Bucharest, Romania

7 Preclinical Department, Apollonia University, Iasi, Romania

*Address all correspondence to: ioannis.mavroudis@gmail.com

References

[1] Espay AJ, Aybek S, Carson A, Edwards MJ, Goldstein LH, Hallett M, et al. Current concepts in diagnosis and treatment of functional neurological disorders. JAMA Neurology. 2018;**75**(9):1132-1141

[2] Perez DL, LaFrance WC, Edwards MJ, Schmid AA, Young J, LaFaver K, et al. Functional neurological disorder: An integrative research agenda for advancing the understanding and treatment of a complex neuropsychiatric disorder. The Lancet Psychiatry. 2021;**8**(2):207-220

[3] Maurer CW, LaFaver K, Ameli R, Hallett M, Horovitz SG. Impaired self-agency in functional movement disorders: A resting-state fMRI study. Neurology. 2020;**95**(18):e2504-e2512

[4] Voon V, Gallea C, Hattori N, Bruno M, Ekanayake V, Hallett M, et al. The involuntary nature of conversion disorder. Neurology. 2016;**86**(17):1614-1620

[5] Carson A, Lehn A, Stone J. Explanatory models in functional neurological disorders. Handbook of Clinical Neurology. 2016;**139**:79-88

[6] Stone J, Warlow C, Sharpe M. The symptom of functional weakness: A paradox of our times. Journal of Neurology, Neurosurgery and Psychiatry. 2010;**81**(3):244-245

[7] Edwards MJ, Adams RA, Brown H, Pareés I, Friston KJ. A Bayesian account of "hysteria". Brain. 2012;**135**(11):3495-3512

[8] Teodoro T, Edwards MJ, Isaacs JD. A unifying theory for functional neurological disorders. Journal of Neurology, Neurosurgery and Psychiatry. 2018;**89**(7):691-692

[9] Voon V, Brezing C, Gallea C, Hallett M. Aberrant supplementary motor complex and limbic activity during motor preparation in motor conversion disorder. Movement Disorders. 2011;**26**(13):2396-2403

[10] Aybek S, Nicholson TR, Zelaya F, O'Daly O, Craig TJ, David AS, et al. Neural correlates of recall of life events in conversion disorder. JAMA Psychiatry. 2015;**72**(1):44-51

[11] Blakemore RL, Sinanaj I, Galli S, Aybek S, Vuilleumier P. Aversive stimuli exacerbate defensive motor behaviour in motor conversion disorder. Neuropsychologia. 2016;**93**(Pt A):229-241

[12] LaFrance WC, Baker GA, Duncan R, Goldstein LH, Reuber M, the NINDS FND Work Group. Minimum requirements for the diagnosis of psychogenic nonepileptic seizures: A staged approach. Epilepsia. 2013;**54**(11):2005-2018

[13] Stone J, Carson A, Sharpe M. Functional symptoms in neurology: Diagnosis and management. Journal of Neurology, Neurosurgery and Psychiatry. 2005;**76**(Suppl. 1):i2-i12

[14] Schrag A, Trimble M, Quinn N, Bhatia K. The syndrome of fixed dystonia: An evaluation of 103 patients. Brain. 2004;**127**(10):2360-2372

[15] Reuber M, Elger CE. Psychogenic nonepileptic seizures: Review and update. Epilepsy and Behavior. 2003;**4**(3):205-216

[16] Baker J, Wyllie E, Dowell T, Paul P, Sandhu M, LaFrance WC. Functional speech and language disorders: Case series and review of literature.

Journal of Neurology, Neurosurgery and Psychiatry. 2017;**88**(12):1092-1098

[17] Ball HA, McWhirter L, Ballard C, Robinson L, Ritchie C, Carson A. Functional cognitive disorder: dementia's blind spot. Brain. 2020;**143**(10):2895-2903

[18] American Psychiatric Association. Diagnostic and Statistical Manual of Mental Disorders (DSM-5). 5th ed. Washington, DC: APA; 2013

[19] Roelofs K, Spinhoven P. Trauma and medically unexplained symptoms: Towards an integration of cognitive and neurobiological accounts. Clinical Psychology Review. 2007;**27**(7):798-820

[20] Edwards MJ, Bhatia KP. Functional (psychogenic) movement disorders: Merging mind and brain. The Lancet Neurology. 2012;**11**(3):250-260

[21] Kleim JA, Jones TA. Principles of experience-dependent neural plasticity: Implications for rehabilitation after brain damage. Journal of Speech, Language, and Hearing Research. 2008;**51**(1):S225-S239

[22] Hebb DO. The Organization of Behavior: A Neuropsychological Theory. New York: Wiley; 1949

[23] Taub E, Uswatte G, Mark VW, Morris DM. The learned nonuse phenomenon: Implications for rehabilitation. Europa Medicophysica. 2006;**42**(3):241-256

[24] Liepert J, Hassa T, Tüscher O, Schmidt R. Motor cortex excitability in patients with functional motor symptoms. Movement Disorders. 2008;**23**(7):1066-1071

[25] Seth AK, Suzuki K, Critchley HD. An interoceptive predictive coding model of conscious presence. Frontiers in Psychology. 2011;**2**:395

[26] Schulz E, Stankewitz A, May A. Neuroimaging of persistent somatoform pain: Structural and functional alterations. Current Rheumatology Reports. 2015;**17**(6):30

[27] Stone J, Hoeritzauer I, Brown K, Carson A. Functional neurological disorder: An update for neurologists. Practical Neurology. 2021;**21**(6): 458-467

[28] Pick S, Goldstein LH, Perez DL, Nicholson TR. Emotional processing in functional neurological disorder: A review, biopsychosocial model and research agenda. Journal of Neurology, Neurosurgery and Psychiatry. 2019;**90**(7):704-711

[29] Nielsen G, Buszewicz M, Edwards MJ, Yardley L. Physiotherapy for functional motor disorders: A consensus recommendation. Journal of Neurology, Neurosurgery and Psychiatry. 2015;**86**(10):1113-1119

[30] Nielsen G, Ricciardi L, Demartini B, Hunter R, Edwards MJ. Outcomes of a 5-day physiotherapy program for functional motor disorder. Neurorehabilitation and Neural Repair. 2021;**35**(2):156-165

[31] Goldstein LH, Chalder T, Chigwedere C, Khondoker MR, Moriarty J, Toone BK, et al. Cognitive–behavioral therapy for psychogenic nonepileptic seizures. Neurology. 2010;**74**(24):1986-1994

[32] Carson A, Stone J, Hibberd C, Murray G, Duncan R, Coleman R, et al. Randomised controlled trial of specialist vs. standardised care for FND. Journal of Neurology, Neurosurgery and Psychiatry. 2012;**83**(3):250-257

[33] Garcin B, Roze E, Mesrati F, Cognat E, Fournier E, Vidailhet M, et al. Transcranial magnetic stimulation as an efficient treatment for functional motor symptom: A proof-of-concept study. Neurology. 2017;**89**(3):291-293

[34] Sitaram R, Ros T, Stoeckel L, Haller S, Scharnowski F, Lewis-Peacock J, et al. Closed-loop brain training: The science of neurofeedback. Nature Reviews Neuroscience. 2017;**18**(2):86-100